Basic Notes in Psychopharmacology

Fourth Edition

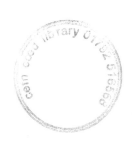

Previous books by the same author

- Levi MI (1987) *MCQs for the MRCPsych Part 1*. Lancaster: MTP Press.
- Levi MI (1988) *MCQs for the MRCPsych Part 2*. Lancaster: Kluwer Academic Publishers.
- Levi MI (1988) *SAQs for the MRCPsych Part 2*. Lancaster: Kluwer Academic Publishers.
- Levi MI (1992) *PMPs for the MRCPsych Part 2*. Lancaster: Kluwer Academic Publishers.
- Levi MI (1996) *Basic Notes in Psychotherapy*. Newbury: Petroc Press.
- Levi MI (1997) *MCQs for the MRCPsych*. Newbury: Petroc Press.
- Levi MI (2005) *Basic Notes in Psychiatry* (4e). Oxford: Radcliffe Publishing.

Basic Notes in Psychopharmacology

Fourth Edition

Dr Michael I Levi MB BS MRCPsych
Consultant Psychiatrist
Bradford District Care Trust
Lynfield Mount Hospital
Bradford, West Yorkshire, UK

Foreword by

Dr Gareth Vincenti
Consultant Psychiatrist & Medical Director
Cygnet Hospital, Harrogate, UK

Radcliffe Publishing
Oxford • New York

Radcliffe Publishing Ltd
18 Marcham Road
Abingdon
Oxon OX14 1AA
United Kingdom

www.radcliffe-oxford.com
Electronic catalogue and worldwide online ordering facility.

First Edition 1993 (published by Kluwer Academic Publishers)
Second Edition 1998 (published by Petroc Press)
Third Edition 2004 (published by Radcliffe Publishing)

New research and clinical experience can result in changes in treatment and drug therapy. Readers of this book should therefore check the most recent product information on any drug they may prescribe to ensure they are complying with the manufacturer's recommendations concerning dosage, the method and duration of administration, and contraindications. Neither the publisher nor the author accept liability for any injury or damage arising from this publication.

British Library Cataloguing in Publication Data

A catalogue record for this book is available from the British Library.

ISBN-13: 978 1 84619 187 9

Typeset by Anne Joshua & Associates, Oxford
Printed and bound by TJI Digital, Padstow, Cornwall

Contents

Section Two: Applied Clinical Psychopharmacology   63

Foreword to the Fourth Edition

For many years the field of psychopharmacology barely changed, but the last 15 years have witnessed a revolution, with new drugs and new treatment strategies following one another in bewildering succession. We now live in the world of guidelines and meta-analyses, and it can sometimes be difficult to see the wood for the trees. Mike Levi's latest edition of his already popular book once again provides the busy clinician with a reliable access point to key essential facts about psychopharmacology.

This fourth edition of *Basic Notes in Psychopharmacology* incorporates a new approach, and contains a large and varied amount of case vignettes and discussion. These illuminate the basic factual text, and provide a useful insight into the clinical approach of an experienced and able clinician. As such, this book will remain invaluable for all training grades within psychiatry, the discerning medical student and our mental health nurse colleagues. Consultants involved in training will also find it of assistance in planning teaching sessions.

This new edition of Mike Levi's book restores the publication to the cutting edge of psychopharmacology and he is to be congratulated on his commitment to the field of psychiatric education.

Dr Gareth Vincenti MB BS LLB FRCPsych
Consultant Psychiatrist & Medical Director
Cygnet Hospital, Harrogate
August 2007

Preface to the Fourth Edition

Following the popularity of the third edition, I was encouraged to write this new edition for junior hospital psychiatrists, general practitioners and medical students.

I have completely updated the book to include new psychotropic drugs that have been launched in the UK since the appearance of the third edition in 2004. I have also reviewed all the drugs covered in the third edition and updated these entries, where appropriate, in the light of current knowledge.

The fourth edition also includes 35 clinical vignettes in the area of general adult psychiatry with suggested psychopharmacological management plans.

MIL
August 2007

Introduction

The purpose of writing this book is twofold: Section One provides a concise summary of psychopharmacology in the form of notes. The drugs discussed in this section of the book are those considered by the author to be the most important drugs that the practising physician needs to know about. The aim is to provide the principal mode of action, indications and adverse effects of the drugs covered. I have based these notes on what is generally regarded to be the most comprehensive textbook[1] for the MRCPsych examination. These notes represent my own view of current clinical practice.

Section Two provides the reader with 35 clinical vignettes in the area of general adult psychiatry with suggested psychopharmaco-logical management plans. I clearly acknowledge the importance of psychosocial treatments in mental illness. However, for the purpose of this book, I am unashamedly focusing on psychopharmacological treatments which play a major part in management.

The reader should study each clinical vignette, consider their answer, then turn the page and see how they got on. Of course, they will not always agree with my suggested psychopharmacological management plan. However, agreement or not is unimportant, as in disagreeing one is forced to justify one's own line of thinking. This can only help to firm up one's own ideas regarding psychopharmaco-logical management.

The book is intended to have wide readership – particularly among junior hospital psychiatrists, general practitioners and medical students. In addition, the book will also be useful to psychiatric nurses, psychiatric social workers, psychiatric occupational therapists and clinical psychologists.

Reference

1 Gelder M, Lopez-Ibor JJ, Andreasen N, eds. *New Oxford Textbook of Psychiatry*. Oxford: Oxford University Press; 2003.

Acknowledgements

The author is indebted to Ms Deborah Barron for her invaluable help in producing the manuscript.

Many thanks also to Dr Gareth Vincenti for his helpful comments and for providing the Foreword to the book.

Basic Psychopharmacology

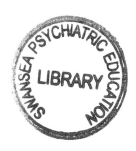

CHAPTER 1

Hypnotic and Anxiolytic Drugs

I BENZODIAZEPINES

(a) Mode of action

1 GABA (γ-aminobutyric acid) agonists; act at benzodiazepine BZ_1- and BZ_2-receptors which are located postsynaptically throughout the brain at GABA-ergic synapses.

2 There are three subtypes of benzodiazepine receptors:
   (i) Omega-1 – mediates hypnotic effect of drug
   (ii) Omega-2 – mediates anxiolytic effect of drug
   (iii) Omega-3 – mediates myorelaxant effect of drug.
   Benzodiazepines act on all three receptor subtypes and therefore have muscle relaxant, anxiolytic and hypnotic effects.

(b) Indications

1 Transient insomnia in those who normally sleep well – if a benzodiazepine is indicated, use one that has a short half-life with little or no hangover effect and only prescribe 1 or 2 doses of the drug, e.g. lormetazepam; dose range 0.5 mg nocte to 1.5 mg nocte.

2 Anxiety disorders (generalised anxiety disorder and panic disorder) – provide symptomatic relief of severe anxiety in the short term (should not be prescribed for more than 2–4 weeks), e.g. diazepam; dose range 2 mg tds increased if necessary to 15–30 mg daily in divided doses. The use of an antidepressant drug should also be considered in this situation (see later).

3 Phobic anxiety disorders – provide some immediate relief of phobic symptoms in the short term.

4 Obsessive compulsive disorders – provide some short-term symp-

tomatic relief (should not be prescribed for more than 2–4 weeks' duration).

5 Acute organic disorder:
- (i) May be used during the night-time to help the patient sleep.
- (ii) In the special case of hepatic failure – may be used during the day-time to calm the patient despite their sedative effects, since they are less likely to precipitate coma – cf haloperidol (which is the usual drug of choice to calm such patients).
- (iii) In the special case of alcohol withdrawal – chlordiazepoxide is the most suitable drug.

6 Chronic organic disorder – may be used to alleviate anxiety.

7 Barbiturate dependence – used to cover the withdrawal symptoms from barbiturates.

8 Acutely disturbed behaviour – if an antipsychotic drug alone fails to bring the situation under control, they may be given in addition a slow intramuscular injection of 2 mg of lorazepam,* if necessary repeated 2 hours later.

9 Akathisia.

(c) Adverse effects

1 Both psychic and physical dependence occur.

2 Chronic benzodiazepine dependence – often manifests features of benzodiazepine intoxication, which are:
- (i) Unsteadiness of gait.
- (ii) Dysarthria.
- (iii) Drowsiness.
- (iv) Nystagmus.

3 Withdrawal effects from benzodiazepines:
- (i) Rebound insomnia.
- (ii) Tremor.
- (iii) Anxiety.
- (iv) Restlessness.
- (v) Appetite disturbance.
- (vi) Weight loss.
- (vii) Sweating.
- (viii) Convulsions.
- (ix) Confusion.
- (x) Toxic psychosis.

* Used but this indication is not currently licensed in the UK.

(xi) A condition resembling delirium tremens.

4 Benzodiazepines – cf barbiturates. Advantages of benzodiaze-pines:

(i) Milder side-effects – including less risk of respiratory depres-sion.

(ii) Less severe physical dependence.

(iii) Less dangerous in overdosage.

(iv) Less likely to interact with other drugs – as induction of hepatic microsomal enzymes does not occur to the same extent.

II BARBITURATES

(a) Mode of action

GABA potentiators; do not act at benzodiazepine receptors; may have specific binding sites elsewhere on the neuronal membrane.

(b) Indications

1 Severe intractable insomnia in patients already taking barbitur-ates – even in such patients, an attempt to slowly withdraw the barbiturate should be considered, covering the withdrawal syn-drome with a benzodiazepine.

2 Dissociative (conversion) disorders – classically, abreaction was brought about by an intravenous injection of small amounts of amylobarbitone sodium. In the resulting state, the patient is encouraged to relive the stressful events that provoked the hysteria, and to express the accompanying emotions. Now, such abreaction can be initiated more safely by a slow intravenous injection of 10 mg of diazepam.

(c) Adverse effects

1 Both psychic and physical dependence occur.

2 Chronic barbiturate dependence – often manifests features of barbiturate intoxication, which are:

(i) Slurred speech.

(ii) Incoherence.

(iii) Dullness.

(iv) Drowsiness.

(v) Nystagmus.

(vi) Depression.

3 Withdrawal effects from barbiturates:

    (i) Clouding of consciousness.
    (ii) Disorientation.
    (iii) Hallucinations.
    (iv) Major seizures.
    (v) Anxiety.
    (vi) Restlessness.
    (vii) Pyrexia.
    (viii) Tremulousness.
    (ix) Insomnia.
    (x) Hypotension.
    (xi) Nausea.
    (xii) Vomiting.
    (xiii) Anorexia.
    (xiv) Twitching.
    (xv) A condition resembling delirium tremens.

4 Drug interactions – induction of hepatic microsomal enzymes leads to increased metabolism of:
    (i) The oral contraceptive pill.
    (ii) Corticosteroids.
    (iii) Warfarin.
    (iv) Tricyclic antidepressants.
    (v) Most antipsychotic drugs.
    (vi) Cyclosporin.
    (vii) Theophylline.

III CHLORAL DERIVATIVES

(a) Mode of action

GABA potentiators.

(b) Indications

Short-term treatment of insomnia, e.g. chloral betaine; rarely used now.

(c) Adverse effects

Abuse potential – therefore should not be prescribed for more than 1–2 weeks' duration.

IV OTHERS

1 CHLORMETHIAZOLE

(a) Mode of action

GABA potentiator.

(b) Indications

In the management of alcohol withdrawal for inpatients only, chlormethiazole may be prescribed in either of two ways:

1 On an as-required basis, i.e. flexibly according to the patient's symptoms.
2 On a reducing regimen basis, i.e. on a fixed 6-hourly regimen of gradually decreasing dosage over 6–9 days.

NB: *The patient must stop drinking when taking chlormethiazole. If chlormethiazole is taken in combination with alcohol, each potentiates the CNS depressant action of the other, and overdosage is frequently fatal; thus nowadays chlordiazepoxide is preferred as an alternative to chlormethiazole in the management of alcohol withdrawal – chlordiazepoxide has the advantage over chlormethiazole of being less addictive and being less dangerous if taken in combination with alcohol.*

(c) Adverse effect

May cause acute cardiac arrest or acute respiratory arrest if taken in combination with alcohol.

2 ß-BLOCKERS

(a) Mode of action

Block ß-adrenoreceptors in the heart, peripheral vasculature, bronchi, liver and pancreas and brain (although CNS penetration is poor).

(b) Indications

Limited use in treating anxiety disorders in which palpitations, sweating or tremor are the most troublesome symptoms, i.e. those anxiety disorders with predominantly somatic symptoms, e.g. propranolol; dose range 40 mg bd (or 80 mg SR) to 40 mg tds.

NB: *ß-Blockers have little effect on subjective feelings of anxiety.*

(c) Adverse effects

Contraindicated in patients with:

1 Asthma.
2 A history of obstructive airways disease.
3 Uncontrolled heart failure.
4 Second- or third-degree heart block.

3 BUSPIRONE

(a) Mode of action

1 Thought to act at specific serotonin ($5HT_{1A}$) presynaptic autoreceptors – as a partial agonist.
2 Response to treatment may take up to 2 weeks – similar to antidepressant drugs.

(b) Indications

1 Short-term treatment (up to several months) of generalised anxiety disorder; usual dose range 5 mg tds to 10 mg tds; maximum dose of 15 mg tds; long-term efficacy is untested.
2 May be useful in the treatment of resistant depression* – as an augmenting agent to SSRIs (by enhancing serotonin accumulation within the synapse).
3 May be useful in the treatment of obsessive compulsive disorder* – as an augmenting agent to SSRIs.

(c) Adverse effects

1 Physical dependence and abuse liability low.
2 Non-toxic augmenting agent, cf lithium carbonate.
3 Does not potentiate the effects of alcohol, cf benzodiazepines, which do.
4 Lacks sedative and myorelaxant properties of benzodiazepines.
5 Contraindicated in pregnancy and epilepsy.

4 ZOPICLONE

(a) Mode of action

1 The first cyclopyrrolone.
2 GABA potentiator – although not a benzodiazepine, it acts on

---

* Used but these indications are not currently licensed in the UK.

benzodiazepine receptors, which are located postsynaptically throughout the brain at GABA-ergic synapses.

3 Acts on Omega-1 and Omega-2 receptor subtypes and therefore has anxiolytic and hypnotic effects.

(b) Indications

1 Transient insomnia in those who normally sleep well – as an alternative to a benzodiazepine; dosage 7.5 mg nocte in adults.
2 For short-term use only (preferably only 1 or 2 doses).

(c) Adverse effects

Since it acts on benzodiazepine receptors, it may give rise to the problems of physical dependence as observed in benzodiazepines if used for long-term treatment.

5 ZOLPIDEM

(a) Mode of action

1 The first imidazopyridine.
2 GABA potentiator – although not a benzodiazepine, it acts on benzodiazepine receptors, which are located postsynaptically throughout the brain at GABA-ergic synapses.
3 Acts on Omega-1 receptor subtype only and therefore has a pure hypnotic effect.

(b) Indications

1 Transient insomnia in those who normally sleep well – as an alternative to a benzodiazepine; dosage 10 mg nocte in adults.
2 For short-term use only (preferably only 1 or 2 doses).

(c) Adverse effect

1 Since it acts on one of the same receptor subtypes as benzodiazepines, it may give rise to the problems of physical dependence as observed in benzodiazepines if used for long-term treatment.
2 May have less abuse potential because it spares the Omega-2 receptor subtype, cf zopiclone.

6 ZALEPLON

(a) Mode of action

Acts on the Omega-1 subtype of the central benzodiazepine's receptor – and therefore has a pure hypnotic effect.

(b) Indications

1 Insomnia (short-term use).
2 Dosage 10 mg at bedtime or after going to bed if difficulty falling asleep; the latter is accounted for by the very short half-life (duration of action) of Zaleplon.

(c) Adverse effect

May have less abuse potential because it spares the Omega-2 receptor subtype, cf zopiclone.

7 PREGABALIN

(a) Mode of action

1 Antiepileptic.
2 Binds to an auxillary subunit (α_2-δ protein) of voltage-gated calcium channels in the central nervous system, potentially displacing [^{3}H]-gabapentin.

(b) Indications

1 Licensed in 2006 for the treatment of generalised anxiety disorder (GAD) in adults.
2 It has been shown to be effective in reducing both the psychological and somatic symptoms of GAD.
3 The dose range is 150 to 600 mg per day given as two or three divided doses. The need for treatment should be reassessed regularly.

(c) Adverse effects

1 Very common side-effects include dizziness and somnolence.
2 Common side-effects include dry mouth, constipation, vomiting and flatulence.

CHAPTER 2

Antipsychotic Drugs

CLASSIFICATION

Conventional antipsychotics

1 Chlorpromazine
2 Haloperidol
3 Trifluoperazine
4 Sulpiride
5 Pimozide
6 Zuclopenthixol acetate

Atypical antipsychotics

1 Risperidone
2 Olanzapine
3 Quetiapine
4 Amisulpride
5 Aripiprazole
6 Zotepine
7 Clozapine

Antipsychotic depot injections

1 Fluphenazine decanoate
2 Flupenthixol decanoate
3 Zuclopenthixol decanoate
4 Haloperidol decanoate
5 Pipotiazine palmitate
6 IM risperidone

CONVENTIONAL ANTIPSYCHOTICS

I CHLORPROMAZINE

(a) Mode of action

1 Dopamine antagonist; blocks D_2-receptors in the mesolimbic cortical bundle – which mediates the antipsychotic action of chlorpromazine.

2 It also has several other biochemical actions which mediate the side-effects of chlorpromazine:
   (i) Dopamine blocking activity at other sites (see later).
   (ii) Antiserotonergic activity.
   (iii) α_1-Adrenergic receptor antagonist.
   (iv) Muscarinic M_1-receptor antagonist.
   (v) Histamine H_1-receptor antagonist.

(b) Indications

1 Schizophrenia:
   (i) Control and maintenance therapy in schizophrenia (usual maintenance dose 50 mg bd to 100 mg tds; maximum dose 1 g daily in divided doses).
   (ii) Chlorpromazine is more sedative and causes fewer extra-pyramidal side-effects, cf haloperidol – thus, chlorpromazine was the drug of choice for schizophrenia (before the advent of atypical antipsychotics).

2 Affective disorders:
   (i) Control of the psychotic components of psychotic depression.
   (ii) Usually brings the symptoms of acute mania under rapid control.

3 Persistent delusional disorder – symptoms are sometimes relieved.

4 Obsessive compulsive disorders – small doses of value when anxiolytic treatment is needed for more than the 2–4 weeks' duration for which benzodiazepines are prescribed.

5 Personality disorders – may be given for short periods at times of unusual stress.

6 Chronic organic disorder – alleviation of certain symptoms of dementia:
   (i) Anxiety.
   (ii) Overactivity.
   (iii) Delusions.

(iv) Hallucinations.

NB: *Care is needed to find the optimal dose; in the elderly there are the special dangers of hypotension, atropinic effects and ECG changes – therefore haloperidol is preferred to chlorpromazine in the elderly.*

   7 Behavioural disturbances – tranquillization and emergency control.
   8 Severe anxiety – short-term adjunctive treatment.
   9 Terminal disease.
  10 Anti-emetic.
  11 Intractable hiccup.

(c) Adverse effects

   1 Extrapyramidal side-effects (EPSEs) – mediated by dopamine-blocking activity at D_2-receptors in the nigrostriatal pathway:
       (i) Acute dystonic reactions.
       (ii) Akathisia.
       (iii) Pseudoparkinsonism.
       (iv) Tardive dyskinesia.
   2 Hyperprolactinaemia – mediated by dopamine-blocking activity at D_2-receptors in the tubero-infundibular system – galactorrhoea in both women and men.
   3 Antiserotonergic side-effect: depression.
   4 Antiadrenergic side-effects (due to blockade of α_1-adrenergic receptor):
       (i) Postural hypotension.
       (ii) Failure of ejaculation.
       (iii) Sedation.
   5 Anticholinergic side-effects (due to blockade of muscarinic M_1-receptors):
       (i) Dry mouth.
       (ii) Blurred vision.
       (iii) Constipation.
       (iv) Urinary retention.
       (v) Tachycardia.
       (vi) Impotence.
       (vii) Exacerbation of glaucoma.
   6 Antihistaminergic side-effect (due to blockade of histamine H_1-receptors): sedation.

NB: *Sedation is mainly mediated through anti-adrenergic activity.*

7 Impaired temperature regulation:
  (i) Hypothermia.
  (ii) Hyperpyrexia.
8 Neuroleptic malignant syndrome (NMS).
9 Bone marrow suppression – leucopenia.
10 Skin photosensitivity and pigmentation.
11 Cardiac arrhythmias.
12 Cholestatic jaundice.
13 Seizures (due to lowering of the convulsive threshold).
14 Weight gain.

II HALOPERIDOL

(a) Mode of action
1 Greater dopamine blocking activity. ⎫
2 Less antiadrenergic activity.   ⎬ cf chlorpromazine
3 Less anticholinergic activity.   ⎭

(b) Indications
1 Mania.
2 Treatment of acute organic disorder during the daytime.
3 Bringing acutely disturbed behaviour under immediate control – since it is less sedative and causes less postural hypotension than chlorpromazine.
4 Other non-affective psychoses.

(c) Adverse effects
1 More EPSE.   ⎫
2 Less sedation.   ⎬ cf chlorpromazine
3 Less postural hypotension.   ⎭
4 Fewer anticholinergic side-effects.
5 NMS.
6 Danger of severe EPSE with haloperidol if a daily dose in excess of 20 mg is combined with lithium carbonate at a serum level of greater than 0.8 mmol/l.
7 ECG changes at high dose – torsade de pointes.
8 Recently the maximum *BNF* recommended dose of haloperidol has been heavily reduced to:
  (i) 30 mg daily in divided doses if taken orally.
  (ii) 18 mg daily in divided doses as an intramuscular injection.
  This is due to EPSE at higher doses.

III TRIFLUOPERAZINE

(a) Mode of action

1 Greater dopamine blocking activity.
2 Less antiadrenergic activity.
3 Less anticholinergic activity.

} cf chlorpromazine

(b) Indications

1 Useful in psychotic patients where sedation is undesirable (i.e. retarded psychotic patients) – since it is less sedative – cf chlorpromazine.
2 Useful in psychotic patients with intractable auditory hallucinations; usual dose range 5 mg bd to 5 mg tds.

(c) Adverse effects

1 More EPSE.
2 Less sedation.
3 Less postural hypotension.
4 Fewer anticholinergic side-effects.

} cf chlorpromazine

IV SULPIRIDE

(a) Mode of action

1 Low doses – thought to block presynaptic dopamine D_3- and D_4-autoreceptors.
2 High doses – blocks postsynaptic dopamine receptors; more specific blocker of D_2-receptors – cf D_1-receptors.

(b) Indications

1 Low doses – may have an alerting effect on schizophrenic patients with negative symptoms such as apathy and social withdrawal (optimum dosage 400 mg bd).
2 High doses – useful in schizophrenic patients with florid positive symptoms such as delusions and hallucinations (optimum dosage 800 mg bd).

(c) Adverse effects

1 Less EPSE – cf chlorpromazine.
2 Less sedation – cf chlorpromazine.
3 Tendency to cause galactorrhoea.

V PIMOZIDE

(a) Mode of action

More specific blocker of D_3- and D_2-receptors – cf chlorpromazine.

(b) Indication

Useful in monosymptomatic delusional psychosis – it is claimed that pimozide has success in specifically targeting monosymptomatic hypochondriacal delusions (dose range 4–16 mg daily).
NB: *Special caution is needed over rate of rise in daily doses.*

(c) Adverse effects

1 Less EPSE. ⎫
2 Less sedation. ⎬ cf chlorpromazine
3 Following reports of sudden unexplained death, CSM recommends:
    (i) An ECG prior to commencing treatment in all patients.
    (ii) ECGs at regular intervals in patients taking over 16 mg daily.
    (iii) A review of the need for pimozide if arrhythmias develop.

VI ZUCLOPENTHIXOL ACETATE

(a) Mode of action

Short-acting injection administered intramuscularly as an oily injection and rapidly released into the bloodstream.

(b) Indications

Useful for immediate management of acutely disturbed behaviour as an alternative to haloperidol since:

1 Zuclopenthixol acetate is more sedative than haloperidol.
2 These injections (maximum of four) are more easily administered to the patient, cf trying to persuade such a patient to comply with regular oral or intramuscular haloperidol.

(c) Cautions

1 Treatment duration should not exceed 2 weeks with a maximum dosage of 150 mg for each injection per 24 hours, and a maximum dosage of 400 mg for each course of injections.
2 Must not be used on neuroleptic-naïve patients, i.e. haloperidol

should have been tried first and been ineffective before considering zuclopenthixol acetate.

ATYPICAL ANTIPSYCHOTICS

I RISPERIDONE

Introduced into the UK in 1993.

(a) Mode of action

1 Potent dopamine D_2-receptor antagonist; in addition it has a regional preference for blocking D_2-receptors in the mesolimbic cortical bundle, cf the nigrostriatal pathway.
2 Potent serotonin $5HT_{2A}$-receptor antagonist.
3 Low affinity for serotonin $5HT_{2C}$-receptors.
4 Potent α_1-adrenergic receptor antagonist.
5 No appreciable affinity for muscarinic M_1-receptors.
6 Low affinity for histamine H_1-receptors.

(b) Indications

1 Treatment of both the positive and negative symptoms of schizophrenia; it appears efficacious in treating both sets of symptoms equally well (usual dose range 4 mg od–6 mg od for maintenance treatment in adults). Treatment of negative symptoms is mediated by blockade of serotonin $5HT_{2A}$-receptors.
2 Alleviation of affective symptoms associated with schizophrenia – mediated by blockade of serotonin $5HT_{2A}$-receptors.
3 Useful in maintenance treatment of schizophrenic patients – it has been given a licence such that it need only be taken once a day to prevent relapse of schizophrenia.
4 Licensed in the UK in 2004 for the treatment of mania in bipolar disorder:
    (i) either as monotherapy or in combination with an antimanic drug (lithium or valproate), no dose adjustment required.
    (ii) co-administration with carbamazapine in bipolar mania not recommended.
    (iii) when initiating treatment, the starting dose is 2 mg od on the first day, which may be increased to 3 mg od on the second day in bipolar mania; due to high affinity for α_1-adrenergic receptors.
    (iv) usual dose range 1 mg od–6 mg od; continued use must be evaluated and justified on an ongoing basis.

5 Some evidence that it may be useful in the treatment of resistant depression* – as an augmenting agent to SSRIs (by enhancing serotonergic accumulation within the synapse).

NB: *Risperidone is available in the UK as an oral preparation (including a quicklet which may be placed on the tongue and allowed to dissolve or dissolved in water); however IM risperidone, a long-acting intramuscular injection form of risperidone, was launched in the UK in 2002 (see later under antipsychotic depot injections).*

(c) Adverse effects

1 Less EPSE (at doses up to and including 6 mg od), cf other anti-psychotic drugs; this benefit may be lost at doses of and over 8 mg od – above this dose, it requires twice daily dosing, i.e. the next increment is 5 mg bd and this may be gradually increased up to a maximum of 8 mg bd.

2 Dose-dependent elevation in prolactin levels, although these are not necessarily related to the possible sexual side-effects.

3 Minimal weight gain due to low affinity for serotonin $5HT_{2c}$-receptors.

4 Postural hypotension – therefore when initiating treatment, the starting dose is 2 mg od on the first day, which may be increased to 4 mg od on the second day in schizophrenia or to 3 mg od on the second day in bipolar mania; both due to high affinity for α_1-adrenergic receptors.

5 No appreciable anticholinergic side-effects.

6 Side-effects include agitation and insomnia due to possible low affinity for histamine H_1-receptors.

7 Some ECG changes (prolongation of the QT_c interval). However, there is no requirement for routine ECG monitoring.

8 Not associated with agranulocytosis.

9 Gastrointestinal side-effects – nausea, dyspepsia, abdominal pain.

10 More akathisia, cf chlorpromazine.

11 Associated with an increased risk of stroke in elderly patients with dementia – thus, the CSM has advised that it should not be used for treating behavioural symptoms of dementia.

* Used but this indication is not currently licensed in the UK.

II OLANZAPINE

Introduced into the UK in 1996.

(a) Mode of action

1 Potent dopamine D_2-receptor antagonist; it preferentially blocks D_2-receptors in the mesolimbic cortical bundle, cf the nigrostriatal pathway.
2 Potent serotonin $5HT_{2A}$-receptor antagonist.
3 High affinity for serotonin $5HT_{2C}$-receptors.
4 Moderate affinity for α_1-adrenergic receptors.
5 High affinity for muscarinic M_1-receptors.
6 High affinity for histamine H_1-receptors.

(b) Indications

1 Treatment of both the positive and negative symptoms of schizophrenia, and affective symptoms associated with schizophrenia (usual dose 10 mg daily; dose range 5–20 mg for maintenance treatment).
2 Maintenance treatment of schizophrenia (once-per-day dosing).
3 Licensed in the UK in 2003 as monotherapy for the treatment of acute mania (starting dose 15 mg daily) and also for the prophylaxis of bipolar affective disorder (starting dose 10 mg daily).
4 It may also be used in combination with an antimanic drug for both the treatment of acute mania and the prophylaxis of bipolar affective disorder (starting dose 10 mg daily).
5 During treatment for acute mania and the prophylaxis of bipolar affective disorder, daily dosage may subsequently be adjusted on the basis of individual clinical status within the range 5–20 mg/day.
6 Some evidence that it may be useful in the treatment of resistant depression* – as an augmenting agent to SSRIs (by enhancing serotonergic accumulation within the synapse).

NB: *Olanzapine is available in the UK as an oral preparation (including a velotab which may be placed on the tongue and allowed to dissolve or dissolved in water); however IM olanzapine, for use in rapid tranquillisation, was launched in the UK in 2004 (see next point).*

7 The rapid tranquillisation of acutely disturbed or violent behaviour in patients with schizophrenia or manic episode, when oral therapy is inappropriate:

* Used but this indication is not currently licensed in the UK.

(i) the recommended initial dose of IM olanzapine is 10 mg.

(ii) a second IM injection, 5–10 mg, may be repeated two hours later.

(iii) the maximum daily dose of IM olanzapine is 20 mg.

(iv) the maximum dose of IM olanzapine is 20 mg in 24 hours on 3 consecutive days.

(v) recently it has been recommended that IM lorazepam can only be administered at a minimum of one hour after the administration of IM olanzapine, cf previously there had been some uncertainty about this as it had been common practice to administer IM lorazepam and IM haloperidol concurrently.

(c) Adverse effects

1 EPSE usually mild and transient if present – responds to dose reduction or to an antimuscarinic drug.

2 Sometimes associated with elevation in prolactin level. However, associated clinical manifestations are rare, cf risperidone.

3 Significant weight gain due to high affinity for serotonin $5HT_{2c}$-receptors; treatment-emergent diabetes mellitus does not appear to be associated with weight gain.

4 Some postural hypotension. However, treatment can be initiated at a therapeutic dose (10 mg daily) without the need to build up from a starting dose; due to moderate affinity for α_1-adrenergic receptors.

5 Anticholinergic side-effects: dry mouth may occur.

6 Side-effects include sedation due to high affinity for histamine H_1-receptors.

7 Not generally associated with clinically significant prolongation of the QT_c interval. No requirement for routine ECG monitoring.

8 Not associated with agranulocytosis.

9 Transient, asymptomatic elevation of hepatic transaminases has been seen in association with olanzapine therapy. However, there is no CSM recommendation to routinely monitor LFTs (liver function tests).

10 Associated with an increased risk of stroke in elderly patients with dementia – thus, the CSM has advised that it should not be used for treating behavioural symptoms of dementia.

III QUETIAPINE

Introduced into the UK in 1997.

(a) Mode of action

1 Weak affinity for dopamine D_2-receptors – similar to clozapine.
2 Low affinity for serotonin $5HT_{2A}$-receptors.
3 Very low affinity for serotonin $5HT_{2C}$-receptors.
4 High affinity for α_1-adrenergic receptors.
5 No appreciable affinity for muscarinic M_1-receptors.
6 High affinity for histamine H_1-receptors.

(b) Indications

1 Treatment of the symptoms of schizophrenia (positive, negative and affective).
2 Maintenance treatment of schizophrenia (twice-per-day dosing; usual dose range 300–450 mg daily in two divided doses for maintenance treatment; maximum 750 mg daily).
3 Licensed in the UK in 2003 for the treatment of acute mania either as monotherapy or in combination with an antimanic drug.

NB: *Quetiapine is currently only available in the UK as an oral preparation.*

(c) Adverse effects

1 EPSE comparable with placebo across the dose range (up to, and including, the maximum dose of 750 mg daily in divided doses in schizophrenia) – the only atypical antipsychotic currently available in the UK with this feature.
2 Prolactin level comparable with placebo across the dose range (up to, and including, the maximum dose).
3 Minimal weight gain due to very low affinity for serotonin $5HT_{2c}$-receptors.
4 Postural hypotension – therefore when initiating treatment in schizophrenia, the starting dose is 50 mg daily in divided doses, which is then increased over six days to 600 mg daily in divided doses in adults; due to high affinity for α_1-adrenergic receptors.

NB: *When initiating treatment in acute mania, the starting dose is 100 mg daily in divided doses, which is then increased over five days to 600 mg daily in divided doses in adults. The maximum dose for acute mania is 800 mg daily in divided doses.*

5 No appreciable anticholinergic side-effects.
6 Side-effects include headaches and somnolence; latter due to high

affinity for histamine H_1-receptors. NB: No increase in somnolence above 100 mg daily as histamine receptors are saturated.

7 Some ECG changes (prolongation of the QT_c interval). However, there is no requirement for routine ECG monitoring.

8 Not associated with agranulocytosis, cf clozapine.

9 Some disturbance in LFTs. However, there is no requirement for the routine monitoring of LFTs.

10 Requires twice daily dosing, cf risperidone (up to 8 mg daily) and olanzapine, which require once daily dosing; this may reduce compliance in patients taking quetiapine for the long-term treatment of schizophrenia.

IV AMISULPRIDE

Introduced into the UK in 1997.

(a) Mode of action

1 Blocks dopamine D_3-receptors (mainly presynaptic) and dopamine D_2-receptors (mainly postsynaptic); limbic selective.

2 No affinity for serotonin $5HT_{2A}$-receptors.

3 No affinity for serotonin $5HT_{2C}$-receptors.

4 No affinity for α_1-adrenergic receptors.

5 No affinity for muscarinic M_1-receptors.

6 No affinity for histamine H_1-receptors.

(b) Indications

1 Treatment of schizophrenic patients with florid positive symptoms or a mixture of positive and negative symptoms (usual dose range 200 mg bd to 400 mg bd; maximum dosage 600 mg bd); it can be initiated at 400 mg bd for florid positive symptoms.

2 Treatment of schizophrenic patients with predominantly negative symptoms (dose range 50 mg to 300 mg daily with an optimum dosage of 100 mg once a day).

NB: *Amisulpride is currently only available in the UK as an oral preparation.*

(c) Adverse effects

1 Lower potential for causing EPSE, cf conventional antipsychotics; however, this benefit is lost at the maximum dosage.

2 Reversible elevation in prolactin level associated with clinical manifestations; not dose dependent and comparable to conventional antipsychotics.

3 Low weight gain due to lack of affinity for serotonin $5HT_{2C}$-receptors.
4 Some postural hypotension. However, treatment can be initiated at a therapeutic dose (200 mg bd for positive symptoms with or without negative symptoms) without the need to build up from a starting dose; due to lack of affinity for α_1-adrenergic receptors.
5 No appreciable anticholinergic side-effects.
6 Side-effects include insomnia, anxiety and agitation.
7 Some ECG changes. However, there is no requirement for routine ECG monitoring.
8 Not associated with agranulocytosis, cf clozapine.
9 There is no requirement for the routine monitoring of LFTs.
10 May be the atypical antipsychotic of choice in patients with diabetes mellitus – due to its lack of affinity for serotonin $5HT_{2C}$-receptors.
11 Requires twice daily dosing, cf risperidone (up to 8 mg daily) and olanzapine, which require once daily dosing; this may reduce compliance in patients taking amisulpride for the long-term treatment of schizophrenia.

V ARIPIPRAZOLE

Introduced into the UK in 2004. Available as an orodispersible tablet in the UK in 2006.

(a) Mode of action

1 Partial agonist at dopamine D_2-receptors:
    (i) Acts as a dopamine D_2-receptor agonist on presynaptic autoreceptors.
    (ii) Acts as a dopamine D_2-receptor antagonist on postsynaptic receptors.
    (iii) Aripiprazole acts as a dopamine system stabiliser in both hypodopaminergic and hyperdopaminergic conditions. As shown in animal models *in vivo*, stabilisation of the dopamine system is proposed to provide antipsychotic efficacy with minimal adverse effects.
2 Partial agonist at serotonin $5HT_{1A}$-receptors.
    (i) May protect against dopamine-mediated adverse effects.
    (ii) May provide anxiolytic activity.
3 High affinity for serotonin $5HT_{2A}$-receptors.
4 Low affinity for serotonin $5HT_{2C}$-receptors.
5 Low affinity for α_1-adrenergic receptors.

6 Low affinity for muscarinic M_1-receptors.
7 Low affinity for histamine H_1-receptors.

(b) Indications

1 Treatment of the positive symptoms of schizophrenia – due to its action as a dopamine D_2-receptor antagonist in the mesolimbic area (where dopamine is excessive).
2 Treatment of the negative symptoms of schizophrenia – due to its action as a dopamine D_2-receptor agonist in the mesocortical area (where dopamine is deficient).

NB: *The usual starting dose is 10–15 mg once daily with a maximum dose of 30 mg daily; aripiprazole is currently only available in the UK as an oral preparation.*

(c) Adverse effects

1 EPSE comparable with placebo.
2 Prolactin level comparable with placebo.
3 Minimum weight gain due to lack of affinity for serotonin $5HT_{2C}$-receptors.
4 Some postural hypotension. However, treatment can be initiated at a therapeutic dose (10–15 mg) without the need to build up from a starting dose; due to low affinity for α_1-adrenergic receptors.
5 No appreciable anticholinergic side-effects.
6 Side-effects include nausea, akathisia, the risk of seizures and insomnia (thus, it is advisable to take it in the morning).
7 Not associated with ECG changes – therefore no requirement for routine ECG monitoring.
8 Not associated with agranulocytosis, cf clozapine.
9 No requirement for the routine monitoring of LFTs.
10 No dose adjustments required in those with renal or hepatic impairment.

VI ZOTEPINE

Introduced into the UK in 1998.

(a) Mode of action

1 Moderate affinity for dopamine D_2-receptors.
2 High affinity for serotonin $5HT_{2A}$-receptors.
3 High affinity for serotonin $5HT_{2C}$-receptors.
4 Low affinity for α_1-adrenergic receptors.

5 Potent noradrenaline reuptake inhibitor.
6 Low affinity for muscarinic M_1-receptors.
7 High affinity for histamine H_1-receptors.

(b) Indications

1 Treatment of the symptoms of schizophrenia – it has a general licence for this, i.e. it is not specifically licensed for any individual set of symptoms (positive, negative or affective). However, it may have antidepressant effects due to its action as a potent noradrenaline reuptake inhibitor.
2 It is initiated in adults at the therapeutic dose of 25 mg tds; if further clinical improvement is required this may be increased to 50 mg tds; it may be further increased to a maximum of 100 mg tds if required.

NB: *Zotepine is currently only available in the UK as an oral preparation.*

(c) Adverse effects

1 May have lower potential for causing EPSE, cf conventional antipsychotics.
2 Sometimes associated with elevation in prolactin levels. However, associated clinical manifestations are rare.
3 Significant weight gain due to high affinity for serotonin $5HT_{2C}$-receptors.
4 Some postural hypotension. However, treatment can be initiated at a therapeutic dose without the need to build up from a starting dose; due to low affinity for α_1-adrenergic receptors.
5 Dry mouth due to potent noradrenaline reuptake inhibition.
6 Side-effects include sedation due to high affinity for histamine H_1-receptors.
7 Other side-effects include asthenia, constipation, tachycardia and seizures.
8 ECG changes (prolongation of the QT_c interval) associated with a possible increased risk of toxicity. In view of this, CSM recommends an ECG prior to commencing treatment in patients at risk of arrythmias. Zotepine should therefore be used with caution in patients with clinically significant cardiac disease.
9 Sometimes associated with neutropenia. Therefore if an infection occurs, a full blood count should be checked.
10 Sometimes associated with elevation in transaminases. Therefore in patients with known hepatic impairment, liver function tests should be monitored weekly for the first three months.

11 Zotepine is uricosuric, therefore it should not be started within three weeks of resolution of an episode of acute gout.

12 Requires dosing three times a day, cf risperidone (up to 8 mg daily) and olanzapine, which require once daily dosing; this may reduce compliance in patients taking zotepine for the long-term treatment of schizophrenia.

VII CLOZAPINE

(a) Mode of action

1 Moderate affinity for dopamine D_2-receptors.
2 More active at dopamine D_4-receptors, cf other antipsychotics.
3 High affinity for serotonin $5HT_{2A}$-receptors.
4 High affinity for serotonin $5HT_{2C}$-receptors.
5 High affinity for α_1-adrenergic receptors.
6 High affinity for muscarinic M_1-receptors.
7 High affinity for muscarinic M_4-receptors.
8 High affinity for histamine H_1-receptors.

(b) Indications

The treatment of schizophrenia in patients unresponsive to, or intolerant of, conventional antipsychotic drugs; at least one drug from two chemically distinct classes should be given a full therapeutic trial before considering clozapine (the atypical antipsychotics may be used as first-line treatment of schizophrenia); in addition, it may be worth considering a course of electroconvulsive therapy (ECT) before starting clozapine therapy, since this can be an effective treatment in resistant schizophrenia (particularly when a significant affective component is present).

NB: *Clozapine treatment must only be instituted by psychiatrists registered with the Clozaril Patient Monitoring Service (CPMS).*

(c) Adverse effects

1 Less EPSE, cf conventional antipsychotics.
2 Asymptomatic rise in serum prolactin.
3 Significant weight gain due to high affinity for serotonin $5HT_{2C}$-receptors; treatment-emergent diabetes mellitus does not appear to be associated with weight gain.
4 Postural hypotension with risk of collapse – therefore treatment should be initiated with a starting dose and then gradually increased over 14–21 days to 300 mg daily in divided doses; usual dose 200–450 mg daily (max 900 mg daily).

5 Anticholinergic side-effects: hypersalivation due to high affinity for muscarinic M_4-receptors in the salivary glands is common; other atropinic side-effects due to muscarinic M_1-receptor blockade also occur.

6 Side-effects include sedation due to high affinity for histamine H_1-receptors.

7 Other side-effects include fits and rare instances of myocarditis.

8 Some ECG changes. However, there is no requirement for routine ECG monitoring.

9 It causes agranulocytosis (life-threatening) in 2–3% of patients taking the drug – its use is therefore restricted to patients registered with the Clozaril Patient Monitoring Service (CPMS) whereby the patient has regular full blood counts to detect any possible agranulocytosis; should this occur, the clozapine must be stopped.

10 No requirement for the routine monitoring of LFTs.

11 Requires twice daily dosing, cf risperidone (up to 8 mg daily) and olanzapine, which require once daily dosing; this may reduce compliance in patients taking clozapine for the long-term treatment of schizophrenia (as may the requirement for regular full blood counts).

ANTIPSYCHOTIC DEPOT INJECTIONS

A IN GENERAL

(a) Mode of action

Long-acting depot injections administered intramuscularly as an oily injection and slowly released into the bloodstream.

(b) Indications

1 For maintenance therapy of schizophrenia – more conveniently given than oral antipsychotic preparations ensuring better patient compliance.

2 For prophylaxis of bipolar affective disorder in patients who have poor compliance with oral prophylactic medication (antimanic drugs) – depot medication certainly protects against hypomanic relapse and some clinicians believe it also protects against a subsequent depressive relapse.

(c) Adverse effects

1 Initially patients should always be given a test dose injection to

ensure that the patient does not experience undue side-effects or any idiosyncratic reactions to the medication or formulation.
2 They may give rise to a higher incidence of EPSE – cf oral antipsychotic preparations.

B MORE SPECIFICALLY

1 Fluphenazine decanoate

(a) Indications

1 Useful in treating agitated or aggressive schizophrenic patients.
2 May be useful for the control of aggressive patients (in view of its sedative nature).

(b) Adverse effect

Contraindicated in severely depressed states – in view of its tendency to cause depression.

2 Flupenthixol decanoate

(a) Indication

Useful in treating retarded or withdrawn schizophrenic patients – in view of its apparent alerting nature.

(b) Adverse effect

Not suitable for the treatment of agitated or aggressive schizophrenic patients – since it can cause over-excitement in such patients in view of its alerting nature.

3 Zuclopenthixol decanoate

(a) Indications

1 Useful in treating agitated or aggressive schizophrenic patients.
2 May be useful for the control of aggressive patients (this specific indication is more clearly established for zuclopenthixol decanoate – cf fluphenazine decanoate) in view of its sedative nature (zuclopenthixol decanoate is more sedative than fluphenazine decanoate).

(b) Adverse effect

Not suitable for the treatment of retarded or withdrawn schizophrenic patients – since it may exacerbate psychomotor retardation in such patients in view of its sedative nature.

4 Haloperidol decanoate

(a) Indication

Maintenance in schizophrenia and other psychosis; usually 4-weekly administration.

5 Pipotiazine palmitate (formerly known as pipothiazine palmitate)

(a) Indication

Maintenance in schizophrenia and other psychosis; 4-weekly administration.

(b) Adverse effect

Allegedly lower EPSE, cf other conventional antipsychotic depot injections.

6 IM risperidone

(a) Indication

1 The world's first ever atypical antipsychotic long-acting intramuscular injection – launched in the UK in 2002.
2 Licensed for the treatment of both the positive and negative symptoms of schizophrenia; it also alleviates affective symptoms associated with schizophrenia; 2-weekly administration.
3 May be the 'depot' (long-acting intramuscular injection) of choice in patients with bipolar affective disorder who are poorly compliant with oral antimanic drugs.*

(b) Adverse effect

Less EPSE, cf other conventional antipsychotic depot injections.

* Used but this indication is not currently licensed in the UK.

CHAPTER 3

Antidepressant Drugs

CLASSIFICATION

Tricyclic antidepressants (TCAs)

1 Amitriptyline
2 Imipramine
3 Dosulepin
4 Trazodone
5 Clomipramine

Monoamine oxidase inhibitors (MAOIs)

Reversible inhibitors of monoamine oxidase type A (RIMAs)

Second-generation antidepressants

1 Lofepramine
2 Mianserin

Selective serotonin reuptake inhibitors (SSRIs)

1 Fluvoxamine
2 Fluoxetine
3 Sertraline
4 Paroxetine
5 Citalopram
6 Escitalopram

Serotonin and noradrenaline reuptake inhibitors (SNRIs)

1 Venlafaxine
2 Duloxetine

Noradrenergic and specific serotonergic antidepressants (NaSSAs)

Noradrenaline reuptake inhibitors (NARIs)

Agomelatine

Pindolol

Thyroxine

I TRICYCLIC ANTIDEPRESSANTS (TCAs)

A IN GENERAL

(a) Mode of action

Monoamine reuptake inhibitors (MARIs) – inhibit the reuptake of both serotonin and noradrenaline into the presynaptic neurone, with the result that both neurotransmitters accumulate within the synapse. Such biochemical changes occur within several hours following administration of the drug, while the antidepressant action of the drug is delayed for about 2 weeks, indicating that some secondary process must be taking place.

(b) Indications

1 Affective disorders:
   (i) Treatment of depressive disorders in the acute stage.
   (ii) Preventing relapse of depressive disorders – need to continue medication for 6 months postclinical recovery after the first episode of a unipolar affective disorder and for several (1–3) years postclinical recovery after 2 or more episodes of a unipolar affective disorder.

NB:

(a) *If the first episode of the depressive disorder is totally destructive to the patient's life, lifelong antidepressant medication should be considered postclinical recovery, as patients cannot afford to have relapses of their disorders.*

(b) *For the last decade or so, the generally held view among informed psychiatrists has been that 'the dose that gets you well is the dose that keeps you well'.*

(c) *TCAs are safer to use in pregnancy where the effects are more clearly established, cf the more recently introduced antidepressants (SSRIs, SNRIs, NaSSAs and NARIs).*

(d) *Antidepressants are non-addictive but are associated with a discontinuation syndrome – therefore they should be gradually withdrawn over a period of 4 weeks (when on the maximum dose), to minimise the risk of discontinuation symptoms.*

2 Anxiety disorders (generalised anxiety disorder and panic disorder) – when medication has to be prolonged beyond the

few (2–4) weeks for which benzodiazepines are prescribed; effective due to their anxiolytic properties.

3 Phobic anxiety disorders – again effective due to their anxiolytic properties.

4 Obsessive compulsive disorders – when anxiolytic treatment has to be prolonged beyond the few (2–4) weeks for which benzodiazepines are prescribed.

NB: *Clomipramine is claimed to have a specific anti-obsessional effect in addition to its anxiolytic effect (see later).*

5 Hypochondriasis – some clinicians advocate a trial of TCAs in all patients (especially if the patient is depressed).

6 Chronic organic disorder with depressive symptoms – a trial of antidepressant medication is worthwhile even in the presence of dementia.

NB: *TCAs tend to increase confusion in the elderly due to anticholinergic side-effects – therefore SSRIs and SNRIs are the preferred antidepressants.*

7 Bulimia nervosa – TCAs produce an immediate reduction in binging and vomiting. However, their long-term effects are less pronounced.

(c) Side-effects

1 Anticholinergic side-effects:
  (i) Dry mouth.
  (ii) Blurred vision.
  (iii) Constipation.
  (iv) Urinary retention.
  (v) Tachycardia.
  (vi) Impotence.
  (vii) Sweating.
  (viii) Confusion.
  (ix) Exacerbation of narrow-angle glaucoma.
2 Cardiovascular side-effects (due to quinidine-like actions):
  (i) Tachycardia.
  (ii) Arrhythmias.
  (iii) Postural hypotension.
  (iv) Syncope.
  (v) Cardiomyopathy.
  (vi) Cardiac failure.
  (vii) ECG changes (e.g. inversion and flattening of T waves).

3 Other side-effects:
- (i) Seizures (due to lowering of the convulsive threshold).
- (ii) Hypomania (in patients with bipolar affective disorder).
- (iii) Tremor.
- (iv) Weight gain.
- (v) Agranulocytosis (uncommon).
- (vi) NMS (rare).
- (vii) Tardive dyskinesia (rare).

(d) Toxic effects (i.e. effects of overdosage)

1 Cardiac arrhythmias/arrest.
2 Prolongation of the QT_c interval.
3 Postural hypotension.
4 Epileptic seizures.
5 Hyperreflexia.
6 Mydriasis.
7 Coma.
8 Death.

B MORE SPECIFICALLY

1 Amitriptyline

(a) Indication

Treatment of agitated depression – in view of its sedative nature:

- (i) Starting dose – 75 mg nocte; build up gradually over 1– 2 weeks to 150 mg nocte (usual dose required for efficacy both in treating the acute stage and for prophylaxis).
- (ii) In patients unresponsive to 150 mg nocte – pushing the dose up to 225 mg nocte or even 300 mg nocte (maximum) may be clinically effective; this would require ECG monitoring, as it is above the *BNF* maximum recommended dose (200 mg nocte).

(b) Adverse effect

Less suitable for the treatment of retarded depression – since it may exacerbate psychomotor retardation in such patients in view of its sedative nature.

2 Imipramine

(a) Indications

1 Treatment of retarded depression – in view of its alerting nature (similar dosage requirements as for amitriptyline – see earlier).
2 Treatment of panic disorders* – imipramine may have a specific effect on autonomic reactivity in panic disorder (where the starting dose is 25 mg).
3 Treatment of phobic anxiety disorders* – some clinicians consider imipramine to be the treatment of choice in agoraphobia.

(b) Adverse effect

Less suitable for the treatment of agitated depression – since it may cause over-excitement in such patients in view of its alerting nature.

3 Dosulepin (formerly known as dothiepin)

(a) Indication

Treatment of agitated depression – in view of its sedative nature:

  (i) Starting dose – 75 mg nocte, increased after 4 days to 150 mg nocte.
 (ii) In patients unresponsive to 150 mg nocte – pushing the dose up to 225 mg nocte may be clinically effective.
(iii) Particularly useful in treating elderly patients – since it has fewer anticholinergic side-effects and fewer cardiovascular side-effects – cf amitriptyline (this also explains why the starting dose of dosulepin can be stepped up more quickly to the therapeutic dose – cf amitriptyline).

(b) Adverse effect

If taken in overdosage, dosulepin is the TCA most commonly responsible for deaths in the UK at present.

4 Trazodone

(a) Mode of action

An antidepressant drug related to the TCAs – but a more selective inhibitor of the reuptake of serotonin, cf amitriptyline and imipramine.

---

* Used but these indications are not currently licensed in the UK.

(b) Indications

1 Treatment of depression with associated anxiety – in view of its sedative nature:
   (i) Starting dose – 150 mg nocte.
   (ii) May be increased to 300 mg daily.
   (iii) Maximum dose of 600 mg daily in divided doses in hospitalised patients (in adults).
2 Very useful in the elderly in the treatment of dementia associated with agitation and aggression* – usually up to 300 mg daily.

(c) Adverse effects

1 Fewer anticholinergic side-effects and fewer cardiovascular side-effects, cf amitriptyline.
2 Safer in overdosage, cf dosulepin.
3 Rarely priapism (discontinue immediately).

5 Clomipramine

(a) Mode of action

Inhibits the reuptake of both serotonin and noradrenaline. However, it is a more selective inhibitor of the reuptake of serotonin, cf the other TCAs.

(b) Indications

1 Treatment of agitated depression – in view of its sedative nature.
2 Treatment of obsessive compulsive disorder – it has been reported that clomipramine has a specific action against obsessional symptoms (owing to it being a more selective reuptake inhibitor of serotonin, cf the other TCAs).
3 Treatment of panic disorder* – it has been reported that clomipramine in low doses has a specific action against panic symptoms (owing to it being a more selective reuptake inhibitor of serotonin, cf the other TCAs).
4 Treatment of phobic states.

(c) Side-effects

It has more anticholinergic side-effects and more cardiovascular side-effects – cf amitriptyline – which may prevent some patients from tolerating it.

---

* Used but these indications are not currently licensed in the UK.

II MONOAMINE OXIDASE INHIBITORS (MAOIs)

(a) Mode of action

Inhibit the enzyme monoamine oxidase which is present in the presynaptic neurone and provides an important pathway for the metabolism of monoamines; thus, MAOIs inhibit the intra-neuronal metabolism of monoamines, resulting in enhanced release of amine neurotransmitters into the synapse.

(b) Indications

1 Treatment of atypical depressive disorders with anxiety, phobic anxiety or obsessional symptoms (i.e. neurotic symptoms).
2 Treatment of resistant depression (particularly tranylcypromine – but it carries a risk of dependence because of its amphetamine-like action).
3 Treatment of panic disorder* – some evidence for usefulness in panic disorder owing to anxiolytic properties.
4 Treatment of phobic anxiety disorders* – reduce agoraphobic symptoms, but there is a high relapse rate when drugs are stopped.

(c) Adverse effects

1 Potentiate the pressor effect of tyramine and dopa present in certain foods (e.g. Chianti wine, cheese spreads, well-hung game, pickled herring, banana skins, broad bean 'pods', Marmite and Bovril).
2 Potentiate the pressor effect of indirect-acting sympathomimetic drugs (e.g. proprietary cough mixtures, nasal decongestants, anaesthetics).

NB: *Both of these types of interaction may cause a dangerous rise in blood pressure ('hypertensive crisis') with fatal consequences; an early warning sign may be a throbbing headache.*

3 TCAs, second-generation antidepressants and SSRIs should not be started until 2 weeks after MAOIs have been stopped in view of the persistence of the effects of MAOIs following discontinuation.
4 MAOIs should not be started until 1 week after TCAs and second-generation antidepressants have been stopped.
5 MAOIs should not be started until 2 weeks after SSRIs have been stopped with the exception of fluoxetine (see below).

* Used but these indications are not currently licensed in the UK.

6 MAOIs should not be started until 5 weeks after fluoxetine has been stopped in view of its long half-life and active metabolite (norfluoxetine).

7 The most commonly prescribed MAOI is phenelzine; however, MAOIs are the least commonly prescribed of the antidepressant drugs because:

   (i) They interact dangerously with certain foods and drugs (see above).

  (ii) The washout period following MAOI discontinuation is 2 weeks – cf the washout period of 1 week following discontinuation of TCAs and second-generation antidepressants (see above).

 (iii) The main indication for MAOIs is atypical depressive disorders (see above), i.e. MAOIs are not generally indicated for endogenous depressive disorders with biological features of depression (except resistant cases when they may be combined with TCAs under specialist supervision).

III REVERSIBLE INHIBITORS OF MONOAMINE OXIDASE TYPE A (RIMAs)

Moclobemide (the first RIMA) was introduced into the UK in 1993.

(a) Mode of action

Selectively and reversibly inhibits monoamine oxidase type A. In contrast, conventional MAOIs inhibit monoamine oxidase types A and B and are irreversible.

  The antidepressant effect of MAOIs is considered to be a result of inhibition of monoamine oxidase type A.

(b) Indications

1 Treatment of endogenous and atypical depressive disorders (dosage: 150–600 mg daily in divided doses; however, there are anecdotal reports of higher doses required for efficacy in endogenous depressive disorders).

2 Treatment of resistant depression (particularly when the patient is unwilling to try a conventional MAOI).

3 Treatment of phobic anxiety disorders (particularly social anxiety disorder).

4 Treatment of panic disorder.*

---

* Used but this indication is not currently licensed in the UK.

(c) Adverse effects

1 Claimed to cause less potentiation of the pressor effect of tyramine and dopa-containing foods, cf conventional MAOIs – however, patients should still avoid consuming large amounts of such foods.
2 Claimed to cause less potentiation of the pressor effect of indirect-acting sympathomimetic drugs, cf conventional MAOIs – however, patients should still avoid such drugs.
3 No treatment-free washout period is required after it has been stopped in view of its short duration of action, cf conventional MAOIs.
4 Should not be started until 1 week after TCAs, second-generation antidepressants and conventional MAOIs have been stopped.
5 Should not be started until 2 weeks after SSRIs have been stopped with the exception of fluoxetine (see below).
6 Should not be started until 5 weeks after fluoxetine has been stopped.
7 Contraindicated in agitated or excited patients – an unfortunate adverse effect since the majority of clinically depressed patients present this way.
8 May precipitate hypomania in patients with bipolar affective disorder.
9 May be the antidepressant of choice in patients with epilepsy.

IV SECOND-GENERATION ANTIDEPRESSANTS

A IN GENERAL

(a) Definition

The next class of antidepressant drugs to be developed after TCAs.

(b) Indications

Particularly useful in the following groups of depressed patients:

1 Patients intolerant of the side-effects of TCAs.
2 Elderly patients.
3 Patients at high risk of suicide.
4 Patients treated in the general practice setting.

(c) Adverse effects

1 Fewer anticholinergic side-effects and fewer cardiovascular side-effects – cf TCAs.
2 Safer in overdosage – cf TCAs.

B MORE SPECIFICALLY

1 Lofepramine

(a) Mode of action

1 Mainly a noradrenergic reuptake inhibitor, i.e. it is a relatively selective reuptake inhibitor of noradrenaline.
2 Structurally a tricyclic antidepressant – however, its adverse effects profile is considerably different from the older 'parent' TCAs (see below).

(b) Indication

Treatment and prophylaxis of retarded depression – in view of its alerting nature (dosage: 70 mg bd; this may be increased to 70 mg mane, 140 mg nocte).

(c) Adverse effects

1 Less suitable for the treatment of agitated depression – since it may cause over-excitement (e.g. sweating, palpitations) in such patients in view of its alerting nature.
2 Much improved side-effects profile – cf older 'parent' TCAs – i.e. lofepramine has fewer anticholinergic side-effects and less cardiotoxicity. Hence, more suitable for use in physically ill patients, cf older 'parent' TCAs.
3 Remarkable record of safety in overdosage – only three deaths recorded to date.
4 May be the antidepressant of choice in pregnancy.

2 Mianserin

(a) Mode of action

1 A presynaptic α_2-autoreceptor antagonist – a novel mode of action for an antidepressant drug with no significant effect on the reuptake of monoamines (i.e. it is only a weak inhibitor of serotonin and noradrenaline reuptake); despite this, it still appears to be an effective antidepressant.
2 Structurally a tetracyclic antidepressant.

(b) Adverse effects

1 No anticholinergic side-effects.
2 Minimal cardiotoxicity – safer in overdosage.   } cf TCAs
3 Rarely causes convulsions – i.e. less proconvulsive.

4 May cause agranulocytosis (particularly in the elderly):
  (i) A full blood count is recommended every 4 weeks during the first 3 months of treatment.
  (ii) If signs of infection develop (e.g. sore throat, fever, stomatitis), treatment should be stopped, a full blood count obtained and subsequent clinical monitoring should continue.
  (iii) This unfortunate side-effect of mianserin together with its questionable efficacy (see mode of action earlier) has limited the prescription of the drug in the hospital setting.

V SELECTIVE SEROTONIN REUPTAKE INHIBITORS (SSRIs) (ALSO KNOWN AS 5HT REUPTAKE INHIBITORS)

A IN GENERAL

(a) Definition

The next class of antidepressant drugs to follow the second-generation antidepressants in time, i.e. SSRIs, are effectively 'third-generation antidepressants'.

(b) Mode of action

SSRIs are highly selective serotonin reuptake inhibitors with little or no effect on noradrenergic processes.

(c) Indications

1 Treatment of depressive disorders, particularly in:
  (i) Patients intolerant of the side-effects of TCAs.
  (ii) Elderly patients.
  (iii) Patients with a high risk of suicide.
  (iv) Patients treated in the general practice setting.
  (v) Patients with cardiovascular disease.
2 Preventing relapse of depressive disorders – need to continue medication for 6 months postclinical recovery after the first episode of a unipolar affective disorder and for several (1–3) years postclinical recovery after 2 or more episodes of a unipolar affective disorder.

NB: *If the patient fails to respond to one SSRI after an adequate trial (i.e. 4–6 weeks at the maximum dose), there is a tendency to try one other SSRI before switching to a different class of antidepressant.*

3 Treatment of panic disorder.
4 Treatment of obsessive compulsive disorder.
5 Treatment of bulimia nervosa.
6 Treatment of post-traumatic stress disorder (PTSD).
7 Treatment of social anxiety disorder.
8 Treatment of generalised anxiety disorder (GAD).
9 Treatment of aggressive behaviour.*
10 Treatment of alcohol dependence – there is some evidence that SSRIs reduce alcohol craving and alcohol consumption in patients with this syndrome.*

(d) Adverse effects

1 No anticholinergic side-effects.
2 No clinically significant cardiovascular side-effects.
3 Safer in overdosage.   cf TCAs
4 More gastrointestinal side-effects (e.g. nausea, vomiting, diarrhoea) which are dose related.
5 More sexual dysfunction (e.g. delayed ejaculation in men, anorgasmia in women).
6 In keeping with good clinical practice, SSRIs should be withdrawn slowly to minimise the risk of discontinuation symptoms.
7 Inhibition of the liver enzyme cytochrome P450 2D6, which is responsible for metabolising the SSRIs and other drugs that might be coprescribed. There is little convincing evidence of clinically significant drug interactions.
8 No clinically significant interaction with alcohol – therefore SSRIs may be prescribed to patients comorbid for alcohol problems and clinical depression.
9 May be less likely to precipitate hypomania in patients with bipolar affective disorder, cf TCAs.
10 May only be prescribed at a therapeutic dose, cf TCAs which have tended to be prescribed at a subtherapeutic dose in the general practice setting.
11 Less likely to cause weight gain, cf TCAs.
12 EPSE (including akathisia) are reported to the Committee on Safety of Medicines (CSM).

---

* Used but these indications are not currently licensed in the UK.

B MORE SPECIFICALLY

1 Fluvoxamine

The first SSRI introduced into the UK, in 1987.

(a) Mode of action

1 Structurally a monocyclic antidepressant.
2 No active metabolite.
3 17–22 hour half-life.

(b) Indications

1 Treatment of depression (starting dose 50 mg nocte to 100 mg nocte; dose range: 50 mg od to 150 mg bd).
2 Treatment of obsessive compulsive disorder (starting dose 50 mg nocte; dose range: 50 mg od to 150 mg bd).

(c) Adverse effects

1 High incidence of nausea and vomiting particularly during the first few days of treatment – this may prevent some patients from tolerating it; such gastrointestinal side-effects may be offset some-what by taking tablets immediately after food and by initiating treatment at a dosage of 50 mg nocte for 1 week and then stepping it up to the usual therapeutic dosage of 50 mg bd (some patients may only respond to the higher therapeutic dosage of 100 mg bd or the even higher dosage of 150 mg bd).
2 Less suitable for patients with hepatic impairment – since it may elevate hepatic enzymes with symptoms.
3 Increases the plasma concentration of theophylline.

2 Fluoxetine

Introduced into the UK in 1989.

(a) Mode of action

1 Structurally a bicyclic antidepressant.
2 Long half-life (2–4 days) with an active metabolite (norfluoxe-tine) which itself has a long half-life with similar activity to the parent compound.

(b) Indications

1 Treatment of depression (dosage: 20 mg mane; this may be increased up to 80 mg mane in adults by gradual 20 mg increments if necessary).

2 Treatment of bulimia nervosa (dosage: 60 mg once daily; maximum dose 80 mg once daily).
3 Treatment of obsessive compulsive disorder – dose range: 20 mg mane to 80 mg mane; increasing the dosage within this range increasingly targets obsessional symptoms.

(c) Adverse effects

1 Less suitable for patients with severe renal impairment – in view of its long half-life and active metabolite.
2 Less suitable for patients with severe weight loss – in view of its catabolic/anorectic nature.
3 Nausea and vomiting appear to be less of a problem with fluoxetine, cf fluvoxamine.
4 Side-effects include sleep disturbances – these may be reduced by taking the fluoxetine in the morning.
5 Increases the plasma concentration of the antiarrhythmic flecainide by cytochrome P450 2D6 inhibition.
6 Other significant drug interactions – increases the plasma concentration of:
   (i) Haloperidol.
   (ii) Clozapine.
   (iii) TCAs.
   (iv) Phenytoin.
   (v) Warfarin.

3 Sertraline

Introduced into the UK in 1990.

(a) Mode of action

1 Structurally different from fluvoxamine, fluoxetine and paroxetine.
2 Has an active metabolite (desmethylsertraline) which has a long half-life with about one eighth of the activity of the parent compound.

(b) Indications

1 Treatment of depression (dose range: 50 mg mane to 200 mg mane).
2 Prevention of relapse in depression and recurrent depression.
3 Treatment of obsessive compulsive disorder (dose range: 50 mg mane to 200 mg mane).

4 Treatment of post-traumatic stress disorder in women only (starting dose 25 mg mane for one week; dose range: 50 mg mane to 200 mg mane).

(c) Adverse effects

1 Side-effects include loose stools and diarrhoea.
2 May have lower potential for drug interactions – since it has no significant interaction with cytochrome P450 2D6.

4 Paroxetine

Introduced into the UK in 1991.

(a) Mode of action

1 Structurally different from fluvoxamine, fluoxetine and sertraline.
2 No active metabolite.
3 24-hour half-life.

(b) Indications

1 Treatment of depression with associated anxiety – the first SSRI to have a licence for this (dosage: 20 mg mane; this may be increased up to 50 mg daily in adults by gradual 10 mg increments if necessary).
2 Treatment of obsessive compulsive disorder (OCD) (dosage: 20 mg mane; this may be increased up to 60 mg daily in adults by weekly 10 mg increments if necessary). It may be the SSRI of choice to treat OCD, owing to its established anxiolytic profile and anti-obsessional effect.
3 The first SSRI to have a licence for the treatment of panic disorder with or without agoraphobia (dosage: 10 mg mane; this may be increased up to 60 mg daily in adults by weekly 10 mg increments if necessary).
4 Prevention of relapse in depression.
5 Prevention of relapse in obsessive compulsive disorder (OCD).
6 Prevention of relapse in panic disorder.
7 Treatment of social anxiety disorder (dosage: 20 mg mane; this may be increased up to 50 mg daily in adults by weekly 10 mg increments if necessary).
8 The first SSRI to have a licence for the treatment of post-traumatic stress disorder (PTSD) (dosage: 20 mg mane; this may be increased

up to 50 mg daily in adults by gradual 10 mg increments if necessary).

9 Treatment of generalised anxiety disorder (GAD) (dosage: 20 mg mane; this may be increased up to 50 mg daily in adults by weekly 10 mg increments if necessary).

(c) Adverse effects

1 Less suitable for the treatment of retarded (anergic) depression – in view of its anxiolytic nature.

2 Nausea and vomiting appear to be less of a problem with paroxetine, cf fluvoxamine.

3 Inhibits its own metabolism by cytochrome P450 2D6 inhibition.

4 Side-effects include a dry mouth and drowsiness.

5 During the initial treatment of panic disorder, there is potential for a worsening of the panic symptoms (hence the starting dose is 10 mg mane, cf 20 mg mane for other indications).

6 When discontinuing paroxetine, it should be gradually reduced by weekly 10 mg decrements to minimise the risk of discontinuation symptoms, i.e. when on the maximum dose of 50 mg daily in adults for depression, this should be gradually withdrawn over a period of 4 weeks.

7 May be the antidepressant of choice in patients wth hepatic impairment.

5 Citalopram

Introduced into the UK in 1995.

(a) Mode of action

1 Structurally different from the other SSRIs.

2 No active metabolite.

(b) Indications

1 Treatment of depression (dosage: 20 mg daily; this may be increased up to 60 mg daily in adults by gradual 20 mg increments if necessary).

2 Prevention of relapse in depression and recurrent depression.

3 Treatment of panic disorder (dosage: 10 mg daily; this may be increased up to 60 mg daily in adults by weekly 10 mg increments if necessary; however, the usual recommended dose is 20–30 mg daily).

(c) Adverse effects

May have lower potential for drug interactions – since it has no significant interaction with cytochrome P450 2D6.

6 Escitalopram

Introduced into the UK in 2002.

(a) Mode of action

1 The *S*-enantiomer of citalopram, i.e. the optical isomer of citalopram with antidepressant activity.
2 More selective than citalopram – which consists of the racemic mixture of both the *S*-enantiomer and the *R*-enantiomer (the latter lacks antidepressant activity).
3 Serotonin transporter theory:
  (i) By removing *R*-citalopram (at the synapse), escitalopram functions more effectively.
  (ii) Escitalopram increases serotonin levels more than citalopram.

(b) Indications

1 Treatment of depression (dosage: 10 mg daily; this may be increased up to 20 mg daily in adults).
2 Treatment of panic disorder with or without agoraphobia (starting dose 5 mg daily for one week; dosage: 10–20 mg daily).
3 Licensed for treatment of social anxiety disorder in 2004 (usual dosage 10 mg daily; dose range 5– 20 mg daily).
4 Licensed for treatment of generalised anxiety disorder (GAD) in 2005 (dosage: 10 mg daily; this may be increased up to 20 mg daily in adults).
5 May be associated with an early symptom relief in the treatment of depression, cf citalopram.
6 Some evidence that it has a superior effect in the treatment of depression, cf citalopram.
7 Some evidence that efficacy in the treatment of depression is comparable to venlafaxine XL, cf other SSRIs where there is considerable evidence that venlafaxine XL is more effective.

(c) Adverse effects

1 Escitalopram has a comparable side-effect profile to citalopram.
2 Co-administration with the known cytochrome P450 isoenzyme CYP2C19 inhibitors omeprazole and high-dose cimetidine, may

require reduction of the escitalopram dose (metabolism of escitalopram is mainly mediated by CYP2C19).

VI SEROTONIN AND NORADRENALINE REUPTAKE INHIBITORS (SNRIs)

1 Venlafaxine

Venlafaxine (the first SNRI) was introduced into the UK in 1995.

Available as a standard formulation requiring twice daily dosing (up to 375 mg daily) and a modified release formulation (XL) to allow once daily dosing (up to 225 mg daily).

(a) Mode of action
1 Structurally a bicyclic antidepressant.
2 It selectively inhibits the reuptake of both serotonin and noradrenaline into the presynaptic neurone (but the predominant effect is on serotonin).
   (i) at low dose (75 mg daily) – its predominant action is on serotonin inhibition, with a lesser action on noradrenaline inhibition.
   (ii) at moderate dose to high dose – it acts more equally as both a serotonin and noradrenaline reuptake inhibitor.

(b) Indications
1 Treatment of depressive disorders (dosage: 75 mg daily; this may be increased to 150 mg daily in major depressive disorder [MDD] and again if necessary to the maximum dose of 225 mg daily for the XL formulation; it may be further increased by 75 mg increments every 2–3 days to a maximum of 375 mg daily in severely depressed or hospitalised patients – this would require twice daily dosing of the standard formulation).
2 There is now considerable evidence that venlafaxine XL is more effective than the SSRIs; however, there is some evidence that the efficacy of escitalopram is comparable to venlafaxine XL.
3 Treatment of moderate to severe generalised anxiety disorder (GAD) (dosage: 75 mg daily in the modified release formulation).

(c) Adverse effects
1 Fewer anticholinergic side-effects.
2 Fewer clinically significant cardiovascular side-effects. } cf TCAs
3 Safer in overdosage.

4 Less likely to cause weight gain, cf TCAs.
5 Gastrointestinal side-effects (e.g. nausea) – these are dose related and occur with a similar prevalence to those observed with SSRIs; they appear to be reduced with the XL formulation.
6 Blood pressure should be monitored in all patients; dose reduction or discontinuation should be considered for patients who experience a sustained increase in blood pressure.
7 May precipitate hypomania in patients with bipolar affective disorder.
8 Frequently reported side-effects are sweating and headache.
9 Drug interactions – potentiation of the anticoagulant effects of warfarin have been reported; should not be used in combination with SSRIs, unless clinically indicated and on the advice of a specialist.
10 For severely depressed or hospitalised patients who require daily doses of 300 mg or more, treatment should be initiated under specialist supervision including shared care arrangements.
11 Should not be used in patients with an identified very high risk of a serious cardiac ventricular arrhythmia.
12 Should not be used in patients with pre-existing uncontrolled hypertension.
13 Should be used with caution in patients with pre-existing heart disease that may increase the risk of ventricular arrhythmias (e.g. recent myocardial infarction).

2 Duloxetine

Introduced into the UK in 2005.

(a) Mode of action

1 It selectively inhibits the reuptake of both serotonin and noradrenaline into the presynaptic neurone. It is a relatively balanced inhibitor of both neurotransmitters, cf venlafaxine where at low dose (75 mg daily) its predominant action is on serotonin inhibition, with a lesser action on noradrenaline inhibition.

NB: *Clinical benefits cannot be inferred from pre-clinical binding studies.*

2 It has no significant affinity for dopaminergic, adrenergic, muscarinic or histaminergic receptors.

(b) Indications

1 Treatment of depressive disorders (dosage: starting and maintenance dose of 60 mg daily; this may be increased to a maximum

dose of 60 mg bd – however, there is no clinical evidence suggesting that patients not responding to 60 mg daily may benefit from dose up-titrations).

2 Provides relief across a broad range of depressive symptoms (both psychological and somatic).

3 Helps to relieve the general aches and pains (GAPs) seen in depressed patients including back pain and shoulder pain.

(c) Adverse effects

1 Most commonly reported adverse effects are nausea, dry mouth and constipation; of the commonly reported adverse effects, the majority are mild-to-moderate and transient.

2 No clinically significant effect on weight.

3 Blood pressure monitoring is recommended in patients with pre-existing heart disease and/or pre-existing hypertension, cf venlafaxine, which should not be used in patients with an identified very high risk of a serious cardiac ventricular arrhythmia and/or pre-existing uncontrolled hypertension.

4 No clinically significant prolongation of the QT_c interval.

5 May be initiated by GPs, cf venlafaxine, which should only be initiated under specialist supervision including shared care arrangements in severely depressed or hospitalised patients who require daily doses of 300 mg or more.

6 Contraindications:
   (i) Hepatic impairment/severe renal impairment.
   (ii) MAOIs.
   (iii) The known cytochrome P450 isoenzyme CYP1A2 inhibitor fluvoxamine.

7 Cautions:
   (i) Bipolar affective disorder/seizures.
   (ii) Other SSRIs/TCAs/venlafaxine.
   (iii) Warfarin.
   (iv) Products that are predominantly metabolised by cytochrome P450 2D6 if they have a narrow therapeutic index.

8 In keeping with good clinical practice, duloxetine should be withdrawn slowly to minimise the risk of discontinuation symptoms.

NB: *The contrasts with venlafaxine are based on the summary of product characteristics (SPC), cf head to head trial data.*

The SPC for duloxetine is based on the clinical trial population at present – although the data set is quite large, it is still not based on naturalistic findings, which will only come out once duloxetine has been on the market for a while, cf venlafaxine, which has been on the market for a long time so many more data have accrued.

VII NORADRENERGIC AND SPECIFIC SEROTONERGIC ANTIDEPRESSANTS (NaSSAs)

Mirtazapine (the first NaSSA) was launched in the UK in 1997 as a conventional tablet.

The world's first ever antidepressant available as an orally disintegrating tablet – launched in the UK in 2003. This soltab formulation should be placed on the tongue and allowed to dissolve, i.e. melt.

(a) Mode of action

1 A presynaptic α_2-autoreceptor antagonist – thus enhancing noradrenergic neurotransmission (like mianserin).
2 A presynaptic α_2-heteroreceptor antagonist – thus preventing the inhibitory effect of noradrenaline on serotonin receptors.
3 A postsynaptic serotonin $5HT_2$- and $5HT_3$-receptor antagonist – thus enhancing serotonergic neurotransmission specifically via serotonin $5HT_1$-postsynaptic receptors.
4 No significant effect on the reuptake of monoamines, cf TCAs, SSRIs and SNRIs.
5 A postsynaptic histamine H_1-receptor antagonist.
6 It has a dual action on both serotonin and noradrenaline from the starting dose (15 mg nocte).

(b) Indications

1 Treatment of depressive disorders (dosage: 15 mg nocte; this may be increased to 30 mg nocte if further clinical improvement is required or if oversedation occurs; it may be further increased to 45 mg nocte if further clinical improvement is required or if less sedation is required).

NB: *Mirtazapine becomes more sedative as the dosage is decreased due to its antihistaminergic effect predominating over its noradrenergic effect. Conversely, it becomes less sedative as the dosage is increased due to its noradrenergic effect predominating over its antihistaminergic effect.*

2 Treatment of resistant depression* – high-dose venlafaxine plus mirtazapine ('Californian rocket fuel') is a combination of anti-

* Used but this indication is not currently licensed in the UK.

depressants with a great degree of theoretical synergy for boosting both serotonin and noradrenaline. As such, it may be useful in the most refractory of depressed patients.

3 Some evidence for treatment of resistant depression in combination with an SSRI* – if there has been a partial response to the SSRI alone after an adequate trial (4–6 weeks at the maximum dosage).

(c) Adverse effects

1 Significantly higher incidence of weight gain, cf placebo – which may be partially due to increased appetite.

2 Significantly higher incidence of drowsiness and excessive sedation, cf placebo – owing to a strong affinity for histamine H_1-receptors.

3 May lack some serotonin-related side-effects – possibly owing to the blockade of serotonin $5HT_2$-receptors, which mediate sexual dysfunction/insomnia/agitation/ anxiety and blockade of serotonin $5HT_3$-receptors, which mediate nausea/vomiting/headache.

4 Lacks cardiovascular side-effects – owing to a very low affinity for α_1-adrenergic receptors.

5 Lacks anticholinergic side-effects – owing to a very low affinity for muscarinic receptors.

6 Blood pressure monitoring is not required, cf venlafaxine XL.

7 There is no clinically significant interaction with warfarin, cf venlafaxine XL.

8 When switching antidepressants, the novel action of mirtazapine reduces the risks of the serotonin syndrome.

9 When switching antidepressants, there is no washout period usually required with mirtazapine, so patient therapy is not interrupted (except for MAOIs).

* Used but this indication is not currently licensed in the UK.

VIII NORADRENALINE REUPTAKE INHIBITORS (NARIs)

Reboxetine (the first NARI) was launched in the UK in 1997.

(a) Mode of action

A highly selective noradrenaline reuptake inhibitor with no significant effect on serotonergic processes.

(b) Indication

Treatment of depression (dosage: 4 mg bd in adults; if further clinical improvement is required, this may be increased to 6 mg mane, 4 mg nocte and again if necessary to the maximum dosage of 6 mg bd in adults).

(c) Adverse effects

1 Anticholinergic side-effects (e.g. dry mouth, constipation).
2 It is not recommended for use in the elderly.
3 When switching antidepressants, the predominantly noradrenergic action of reboxetine reduces the risk of serotonin syndrome.
4 When switching antidepressants, there is no washout period usually required with reboxetine, so patient therapy is not interrupted (except for MAOIs).

IX AGOMELATINE*

(a) Mode of action

1 The first melatonergic antidepressant – an agonist at melatonin MT_1 and MT_2 receptors.
2 A specific antagonist at $5HT_{2C}$ receptors – increases noradrenaline and dopamine levels due to $5HT_{2C}$ blockade.
3 No effect on serotonin levels.

(b) Indication**

Treatment of major depressive disorder (MDD) – starting dose 25 mg nocte; this may be increased to 50 mg nocte if further clinical improvement is required.

---

* Due to be launched in the UK in 2008.
** Used but this indication is not currently licensed in the UK.

(c) Adverse effects

1 May be sleep promoting – possibly owing to the affinity for melatonin MT_1 and MT_2 receptors, and the blockade of $5HT_{2C}$ receptors.
2 Reduced sexual dysfunction – possibly owing to the blockade of $5HT_{2C}$ receptors.
3 Lack of discontinuation symptoms, cf paroxetine.
4 No weight gain – weight neutral.
5 No prolongation of the QT_c interval.
6 Frequent side-effects include headache, nausea and dizziness.
7 Cytochrome P450 1A2 is the main route for metabolism – do not use in severe hepatic impairment.
8 No dose adjustment required in those with renal impairment.

X PINDOLOL

(a) Indications*

1 Some evidence for treatment of resistant depression as an augmenting agent to SSRIs (by enhancing serotonergic accumulation within the synapse).
2 Some evidence for treatment of resistant depression as part of the triple therapy:
    (i) SSRI.
    (ii) Buspirone.
    (iii) Pindolol.

XI THYROXINE

(a) Indications*

1 It may be used to augment antidepressant drug treatment in resistant depression.
2 It may have mood-elevating properties when clinical depression and subclinical hypothyroidism co-exist (the latter being defined as a free thyroxine serum level at the lower end of the normal range).

---

* Used but these indications are not currently licensed in the UK.

CHAPTER 4

Antimanic Drugs

I LITHIUM CARBONATE

(a) Mode of action

The precise mechanism by which lithium produces its therapeutic effect is complex and poorly understood.

Postulated mechanisms of therapeutic effects:

1 Decreased neurotransmitter postsynaptic receptor sensitivity.
2 Stimulates exit of Na^+ from cells where intracellular Na^+ is elevated (as in depression) by stimulating the Na^+/K^+ pump mechanism.
3 Stimulates entry of Na^+ into cells where intracellular Na^+ is reduced (as in mania).
4 Influences Ca^{2+} and Na^+ transfer across cell membranes including the Ca^{2+}-dependent release of neurotransmitter.
5 Inhibits both cyclic AMP and inositol phosphate 'second messenger' systems in the membrane – this mechanism mediates the long-term side-effects of nephrogenic diabetes insipidus and hypothyroidism (see below), i.e. lithium blocks ADH-sensitive adenyl cyclase and TSH-sensitive adenyl cyclase, respectively.
6 Interacts with Ca^{2+} and Mg^{2+}, thereby increasing cell membrane permeability.

(b) Indications

1 Treatment of depressive disorders:
   (i) Treatment can be justified in the acute stages of depressive disorders, when other measures have failed.
   (ii) Treatment of resistant depression – i.e. effective in patients who have failed to respond to a cyclic antidepressant drug (mono-, bi-, tri-or tetracyclic antidepressants).

(iii) Enhances the effects of TCAs and MAOIs.

(iv) Enhances the effects of SSRIs – however, lithium should be introduced cautiously because of the risk of the serotonin syndrome developing (owing to enhanced serotonergic activity); this risk appears to be lowest with fluvoxamine.

2 Preventing relapse of depressive disorders:

(i) In unipolar affective disorders:

- Lithium reduces the rate of relapse (but is probably no more effective than continuing TCA treatment).
- After the first episode, treatment should be prolonged for 6 months postclinical recovery.
- After 2 or more episodes – treatment should be prolonged for several (1–3) years post-clinical recovery; lithium is particularly useful in the prophylaxis of recurrent uni-polar depression.
- Continuing treatment with lithium reduces the rate of relapse after treatment with ECT.

(ii) In bipolar affective disorders – prolonged administration of lithium (5 years) prevents relapses into depression.

3 Treatment of mania: Lithium is effective in high doses (1000 mg nocte), but the therapeutic response usually only occurs in the second week of treatment; thus, the response to lithium is slower than the response to antipsychotic drugs.

4 Preventing relapse of mania: In bipolar affective disorders, pro-longed administration of lithium (5 years) prevents relapses into mania.

5 Treatment of mixed affective states.

6 Prophylaxis of schizoaffective disorders – in combination with an antipsychotic depot injection.

7 Treatment of aggressive or self-mutilating behaviour.

(c) Adverse effects

1 Short-term side-effects:

(i) Gastrointestinal disturbances (nausea, vomiting, diar-rhoea).

(ii) Fine tremor.

(iii) Muscle weakness.

(iv) Polyuria.

(v) Polydypsia.

2 Long-term side-effects:

(i) Nephrogenic diabetes insipidus.

 (ii) Hypothyroidism.
 (iii) Cardiotoxicity.
 (iv) Irreversible renal damage (in patients with pre-existing renal pathology).
 (v) Oedema.
 (vi) Weight gain.
 (vii) Tardive dyskinesia and other movement disorders.
3 Toxic effects:
 (i) Increasing gastrointestinal disturbances (anorexia, vomiting, diarrhoea).
 (ii) Increasing CNS disturbances (coarse tremor, drowsiness, ataxia, nystagmus, incoordination, slurring of speech, convulsions, coma).
 (iii) The effects of lithium overdosage may be fatal – hence it is important that the serum lithium level be closely monitored to ensure that it lies within the therapeutic range of 0.4–1.0 mmol/l (the lower end of this range is for maintenance therapy; the higher end of this range is for treatment in the acute stages of illness) in blood samples taken 12 hours after the last dose of lithium; serum lithium levels over 1.5 mmol/l may be fatal.
 (iv) Once stabilized on lithium carbonate, the following should be monitored:
 • Every 3 months – serum lithium level and serum urea and electrolytes.
 • Every 6 months – thyroid functions test.
 • Every 12 months – ECG.

NB: *Before commencing lithium therapy, baseline investigations should include a serum urea and electrolytes, a thyroid function test and an ECG.*

4 Drug interactions:
 (i) Sodium depletion raises the serum lithium level and may result in lithium toxicity – therefore the concurrent use of diuretics (particularly thiazides) should be avoided.
 (ii) The concurrent use of carbamazepine with lithium may result in neurotoxicity without raising the serum lithium level – hence if carbamazepine is added to lithium, it should be done so with caution – cf the concurrent use of sodium valproate with lithium, which is safe.
 (iii) NSAIDs raise the serum lithium level and may result in

lithium toxicity – therefore their concurrent use with lithium should be avoided.

(iv) ACE inhibitors raise the serum lithium level.

5 Contraindications:

(i) Pregnancy.

(ii) Breast feeding.

(iii) Renal impairment.

II CARBAMAZEPINE

Available as a standard formulation requiring three times a day dosing, and a modified-release formulation (Tegretol Retard) to allow twice daily dosing (up to 800 mg bd).

(a) Mode of action

1 Structurally similar to the tricyclic antidepressant imipramine – however, carbamazepine has no effect on monoamine reuptake.

2 Thought to mediate its therapeutic effect by inhibiting kindling phenomena in the limbic system.

(b) Indications

1 Treatment of depressive disorders:*

(i) Treatment of resistant depression, i.e. worth a trial in patients who have failed to respond to a cyclic anti-depressant drug and lithium carbonate.

(ii) Enhances the effects of TCAs and SSRIs.

2 Preventing relapse of depressive disorders:

(i) It prevents relapses into depression in both recurrent uni-polar affective disorders and recurrent bipolar affective disorders.

(ii) It is the mood stabiliser of choice in patients with both epilepsy and bipolar affective disorder since it also has anticonvulsant properties.

3 Treatment of mania* – carbamazepine is effective in high doses (600 mg bd–800 mg bd), but the therapeutic response usually only occurs in the second week of treatment; thus, the response to carbamazepine is slower than the response to antipsychotic drugs.

4 Preventing relapse of mania:

(i) In patients who fail to respond to lithium carbonate – carbamazepine can either be substituted for, or added to,

* Used but these indications are not currently licensed in the UK.

lithium; the two drugs appear to have a synergistic effect when used in combination (but see earlier note on their concurrent use).

    (ii) In patients with the rapid-cycling form of bipolar affective disorder (i.e. four or more affective episodes per year) – carbamazepine is a better prophylactic agent than lithium carbonate.

5 Treatment of all forms of epilepsy – except absence seizures.
6 Treatment of trigeminal neuralgia.
7 Treatment of behavioural disorders secondary to limbic epileptic instability.*
8 Treatment of aggressive behaviour (including after head injury).*
9 Treatment of acute alcohol withdrawal.*

(c) Adverse effects

1 Side-effects:
    (i) Dizziness and drowsiness.
    (ii) Generalised erythematous rash (3%).
    (iii) Visual disturbances (especially double vision).
    (iv) Gastrointestinal disturbances (anorexia, constipation).
    (v) Leucopenia and other blood disorders.
    (vi) Hyponatraemia.

2 Carbamazepine should be initiated at a dosage of 200 mg bd (due to autoinduction, i.e. it often raises the serum level of an active metabolite of carbamazepine) and increased after 1 week to the usual therapeutic dosage of 200 mg mane, 400 mg nocte required for prophylaxis (some patients may require 400 mg bd) – carbamazepine is a less toxic drug than lithium carbonate and regular serum level estimation appears to be unnecessary; however, because of the slight risk of leucopenia and other blood disorders, it is important that full blood count is monitored periodically.

3 Carbamazepine is an inducer of the liver enzyme cytochrome P450 2D6 – thus it can lower plasma haloperidol levels by half.

4 Carbamazepine also decreases the plasma concentration of:
    (i) Oral contraceptives.
    (ii) Warfarin.

5 The plasma concentration of carbamazepine is increased by:
    (i) Erythromycin.
    (ii) Cimetidine.

* Used but these indications are not currently licensed in the UK.

(iii) Calcium-channel blockers.

(iv) Isoniazid.

6 The plasma concentration of carbamazepine is reduced by:
   Phenytoin.

NB: *The maximum dosage of carbamazepine is 800 mg bd (prescribed as Tegretol Retard).*

III SODIUM VALPROATE/ VALPROATE SEMISODIUM

Sodium valproate is available as a standard formulation requiring three times a day dosing, and a modified-release formulation (Epilim Chrono) to allow twice daily dosing (maximum of 2.5 g daily in divided doses).

NB: *Valproate semisodium (comprising equimolar amounts of sodium valproate and valproic acid) is currently licensed in the UK and USA for bipolar affective disorder. Sodium valproate has also been used, but it is unlicensed for this indication. In terms of cost, valproate semisodium is more expensive than sodium valproate (prescribed as Epilim Chrono) for equivalent dosages.*

(a) Mode of action

1 Sodium valproate is thought to mediate its therapeutic effect through indirect effects on GABA-ergic systems (i.e. it may slow GABA breakdown by inhibiting succinic semialdehyde dehydrogenase), implying a possible underlying biochemical disturbance of GABA deficiency in some affective disorders.

2 Valproate semisodium is thought to permeate the blood–brain barrier more easily, cf sodium valproate – this, in turn, results in a higher concentration of valproate in the brain with valproate semisodium, cf an equivalent dose of sodium valproate.

(b) Indications

1 Treatment of depressive disorders:*
   (i) Treatment of resistant depression, i.e. worth a trial in patients who have failed to respond to a cyclic antidepressant drug, lithium carbonate and carbamazepine.
   (ii) Enhances the effects of TCAs and SSRIs.

---

* Used but this indication is not currently licensed in the UK.

2 Preventing relapse of depressive disorders* – they prevent relapses into depression in bipolar affective disorders.

3 Treatment of mania – sodium valproate is effective in high doses (600 mg bd – 1200 mg bd), but the therapeutic response usually only occurs in the second week of treatment; thus, the response to sodium valproate is slower than the response to antipsychotic drugs.

NB: *With valproate semisodium, the therapeutic response is claimed to occur in the first week of treatment, cf sodium valproate [the dosing for valproate semisodium is 750 mg daily in divided doses (day one), then 500 mg bd to 1000 mg bd or 20 mg/kg/day from day two onwards].*

4 Preventing relapse of mania:*
   (i) Effective as an antimanic drug in some manic patients who fail to respond to lithium carbonate and carbamazepine.
   (ii) In the case of lithium carbonate, sodium valproate can be safely added to it and has been shown to enhance the effectiveness of lithium as an antimanic drug.
   (iii) May also be used as a first-line treatment – on both clinical and litigation grounds, valproate semisodium should be preferred to sodium valproate.

5 Treatment of all forms of epilepsy.

NB: *It is better to prescribe valproate semisodium as the brand Depakote, to avoid confusion with sodium valproate.*

(c) Adverse effects

1 Side-effects:
   (i) Recent concern over severe hepatic and pancreatic toxicity.
   (ii) Haematological disturbance (thrombocytopenia, inhibition of platelet aggregation).
   (iii) Drowsiness, weight gain and hair loss.

2 Sodium valproate is initiated at a dosage of 200 mg bd and increased after 1 week to 400 mg bd and again after another week to 600 mg bd, the usual therapeutic dosage required for prophylaxis (some patients may require 800 mg bd) – sodium valproate is a less toxic drug than lithium and regular serum level estimation appears to be unnecessary; however, because of the slight risk of severe hepatic toxicity, severe pancreatic toxicity and haematological disturbance of platelet function, it is important

---

* Used but these indications are not currently licensed in the UK.

that liver function tests, serum amylase level and full blood count are monitored periodically.

NB: *The maximum dosage of sodium valproate is 2.5 g daily in divided doses (prescribed as Epilim Chrono).*

Applied Clinical Psychopharmacology

20 BIPOLAR AFFECTIVE DISORDER (DEPRESSION) – BIPOLAR DEPRESSION

21 BIPOLAR AFFECTIVE DISORDER (ACUTE MANIA) IN PREGNANCY

22 NON-RESISTANT SCHIZOPHRENIA

23 RESISTANT SCHIZOPHRENIA

24 SCHIZOPHRENIA WITH NEGATIVE SYMPTOMS

25 SCHIZOPHRENIFORM PSYCHOSIS IN A PATIENT WITH EPILEPSY

26 SCHIZOPHRENIA IN PREGNANCY

27 SCHIZOAFFECTIVE DISORDER (SCHIZOMANIA)

28 ACUTE ORGANIC DISORDER

29 ALZHEIMER'S DISEASE (MILD TO MODERATE)

30 ANOREXIA NERVOSA

31 ACUTE ALCOHOL WITHDRAWAL/ALCOHOL DEPENDENCE

32 ACUTE OPIATE WITHDRAWAL/CHRONIC OPIATE DEPENDENCE

33 ACUTE BENZODIAZEPINE WITHDRAWAL/CHRONIC BENZODIAZEPINE DEPENDENCE

34 SELF-INJURIOUS BEHAVIOUR (SIB)/LEARNING DISABILITY/ TEMPORAL LOBE EPILEPSY

35 THE ACUTELY DISTURBED PATIENT – RAPID TRANQUILLISATION

QUESTION 1

BORDERLINE PERSONALITY DISORDER (BPD)

- A 26-year-old Caucasian woman.
- She was admitted to the medical ward of the local district general hospital following an overdose of 12 **paracetamol** tablets as a result of a recent break-up with her boyfriend whom she attacked violently prior to admission.
- Five-year history of taking similar overdoses in the setting of unstable relationships, which usually result in her being discharged from the medical ward, but occasionally result in her being admitted to the acute psychiatric unit at her own request. On this occasion it was also decided to admit her to the acute psychiatric unit, which she felt she needed. She has remained there as an inpatient for the last seven days.
- She has been observed to have affective instability throughout this period. She has exhibited undue anger, variable moods, chronic boredom, doubts about her personal identity and intolerance of being left alone. She has also exhibited transient stress-related psychotic symptoms, impulsive behaviour that is damaging to herself and suicidal and self-harming behaviours. In addition, she has violently attacked nursing staff on the ward.
- Her current medication is **haloperidol** 5 mg tds.
- The working diagnosis is that of a borderline personality disorder (BPD).

What is the psychopharmacological management of this patient?

ANSWER 1

BORDERLINE PERSONALITY DISORDER (BPD)

- Admission to hospital should be avoided whenever possible in such a patient, but may be necessary for short periods of crisis.
- The management plan aims to bring about limited changes in the patient's circumstances so that she has less contact with situations which provoke her difficulties and more opportunity to develop the assets in her personality.
- Several of the features of her BPD may be expected intuitively to respond to psychopharmacological intervention. These features include affective instability, impulsive behaviour that is damaging to herself, transient stress-related psychotic symptoms and suicidal and self-harming behaviours.
- Psychopharmacological intervention is often used during the short periods of crisis when admission to hospital is clinically indicated. During these periods the clinical features of her BPD can be severe, distressing and potentially even life-threatening.
- She is currently taking the conventional antipsychotic **haloperidol** 5 mg tds. She has continued to display aggressive and self-harming behaviour with this medication despite taking it for seven days at the maximum recommended dose for acutely disturbed behaviour. Therefore, it is worth considering switching her antipsychotic to the atypical antipsychotic **olanzapine**, which seems to be effective in reducing both aggression and self-harming behaviour in BPD.
- If she continues to display impulsivity and aggressiveness consider adding in an antidepressant from the selective serotonin reuptake inhibitor (SSRI) class of antidepressants. **Citalopram** would be a suitable choice of an SSRI. The SSRIs have been shown to reduce impulsivity and aggression in BPD. SSRIs may exacerbate anxiety and agitation in the short term; however, these symptoms may be reduced with a short-term course of benzodiazepines.
- If she continues to display anger, aggression and impulsivity, consider adding in an antimanic drug. Up to 50% of patients with BPD may also have a bipolar spectrum disorder and antimanic drugs are therefore commonly prescribed to such patients. **Valproate semisodium** would be a suitable choice – it has been shown to reduce anger, aggression and impulsivity in BPD.
- Whether or not long-term psychopharmacological intervention is indicated in a patient such as this remains contentious.

QUESTION 2

PANIC DISORDER

- A 32-year-old Caucasian man.
- Admitted to hospital (after a domiciliary visit by his general practitioner) with shaking, the sensation of feeling smothered, the feeling of choking, chest pain, nausea, feeling dizzy and de-realisation. He was terrified by this episode and had a fear of dying.
- On admission, he did not admit to any biological features of depression or to any psychotic symptoms. He also did not admit to any alcohol or illicit drug abuse, or excessive use of caffeine.
- He exhibited palpitations, sweating, trembling and shortness of breath. He also exhibited obsessional symptoms, but they did not dominate the clinical picture.
- There was a long history of panic disorder with panic attacks; that is, various combinations of psychological and physical manifestation of anxiety not attributable to real danger and occurring in attacks. He had been admitted to hospital for this on four previous occasions, his last admission being some three years earlier, when he responded well to the selective serotonin reuptake inhibitor (SSRI) **citalopram** 60 mg mane. He has continued to comply with this medication.
- The working diagnosis is that of a relapse of his panic disorder.

What is the psychopharmacological management of this patient?

ANSWER 2

PANIC DISORDER

- Selective serotonin reuptake inhibitors (SSRIs) are now considered to be first-line drug treatment in the management of panic disorder.
- The patient has previously responded well, and been well maintained on the SSRI **citalopram** 60 mg mane (the maximum dose). Unfortunately, however, he has experienced a relapse of his panic disorder despite complying with this medication. There is also no scope for increasing the dosage of the **citalopram** since it is already at the maximum dosage.
- In this respect, it is worth considering a switch to a second SSRI before abandoning this class of antidepressant. A good choice for such a second SSRI would be **escitalopram**. Like **citalopram**, this is also licensed for the treatment of panic disorder. **Escitalopram** is a more selective serotonin reuptake inhibitor than **citalopram** and is thought to function more effectively than **citalopram**, according to the serotonin transporter theory (this theory will be explained later in the answer to the clinical vignette on depression with panic attacks). The starting dose for **escitalopram** in panic disorder is 5 mg daily for one week; the dose range is 10 mg to 20 mg daily.
- If the patient fails to respond to the second SSRI **escitalopram,** consider switching to a different class of antidepressant. The tricyclic antidepressants (TCAs)* may be considered as the next antidepressant class of choice in the treatment of panic disorder based on standard NICE clinical guidelines and on local trust clinical guidelines. From among the TCAs, **clomipramine*** may be considered as a good choice in this patient – it has been reported that **clomipramine** in low doses has a specific action against panic symptoms (owing to its being a more selective reuptake inhibitor of serotonin, cf the other TCAs).
- If the patient fails to respond to the TCA **clomipramine,** consider switching to the reversible inhibitor of monoamine-oxidase type A (RIMA) **moclobemide.*** Like conventional monoamine-oxidase inhibitors (MAOIs),* it has also been used in the treatment of panic disorder. However, **moclobemide** has fewer concerns regarding its dietary restrictions, cf conventional MAOIs.

* Used but these indications are not currently licensed in the UK.

QUESTION 3

OBSESSIVE COMPULSIVE DISORDER (OCD)

- A 32-year-old Caucasian man.
- Following an outpatient consultation with his consultant psychiatrist, admitted to hospital with obsessional thoughts in the form of repeated and intrusive words, which were upsetting to him and of a violent and sexual theme. He also had obsessional ruminations in the form of repeated worrying themes about the world ending.
- On admission, he did not admit to any biological features of depression or to any psychotic symptoms. He also did not admit to any alcohol or illicit drug abuse.
- He exhibited obsessional doubts in the form of repeated themes expressing uncertainty about whether or not he had turned off a gas tap that might cause a fire. He also exhibited obsessional slowness as a result of his obsessional doubts.
- There was a long history of obsessive compulsive disorder (OCD) with obsessions and compulsive rituals (the motor component of obsessional thoughts), that is, obsessions similar to those he presented with on this occasion and compulsive rituals that are usually associated with obsessions, as if they have the function of reducing the distress caused by the obsessions. He had been admitted to hospital for his OCD on four previous occasions, his last admission being some three years earlier, when he responded well to **fluoxetine** 60 mg mane. He has continued to comply with this medication.
- A working diagnosis is that of a relapse of his OCD.

What is the psychopharmacological management of this patient?

ANSWER 3

OBSESSIVE COMPULSIVE DISORDER (OCD)

- The selective serotonin reuptake inhibitors (SSRIs) are now considered to be first-line drug treatments in the management of OCD.
- The patient has previously responded well, and has been well maintained on the SSRI **fluoxetine** 60 mg mane. Unfortunately, however, he has experienced a relapse of his OCD despite complying with his medication. However, there is scope for increasing the dosage of the **fluoxetine** to 80 mg mane (the maximum dose), which may lead to successful clinical remission of the patient's symptoms.
- If the patient fails to respond to **fluoxetine** 80 mg mane, it is worth considering a switch to a second SSRI before abandoning this class of antidepressant. A good choice for such a second SSRI would be **sertraline**. High-dose **sertraline** is often needed in OCD, i.e. 150 mg to 200 mg daily. Like **fluoxetine**, this is also licensed for the treatment of OCD. It may be preferred to the two other SSRIs licensed for OCD, namely **fluvoxamine** and **paroxetine.** This is because of the association of a high incidence of nausea and vomiting with **fluvoxamine**, and because of the possible association of a higher risk of discontinuation symptoms with **paroxetine**, cf the other SSRIs.
- If the patient fails to respond to the second SSRI **sertraline**, consider switching to a different class of antidepressant. The tricyclic antidepressants (TCAs) may be considered as the next antidepressant class of choice in the treatment of OCD, based on standard NICE clinical guidelines and on local trust clinical guidelines. From the TCAs, **clomipramine** may be considered as the drug of choice in this patient – it has been reported that **clomipramine** has a specific action against obsessional symptoms (owing to its being a more selective reuptake inhibitor of serotonin, cf the other TCAs). The likely dose of **clomipramine** is 100 mg to 150 mg daily, but this will need to be built up slowly because of side-effects. It is also the only TCA licensed for the treatment of obsessional states.
- The addition of **buspirone** and/or anti-psychotic drugs may help improve a suboptimal response to antidepressants.
- The response times to antidepressants are slower in OCD than depression.

QUESTION 4

POST-TRAUMATIC STRESS DISORDER (PTSD)

- A 28-year-old Caucasian woman.
- Admitted to the psychiatric unit of the local district general hospital after a recent road traffic accident (RTA), having initially been assessed in the Accident and Emergency Department of the same hospital.
- On admission, she admitted to having been exposed to an RTA two months earlier. At the time of the RTA she was assessed in the same Accident and Emergency Department. She did not sustain any significant physical injuries and was subsequently sent home. She admitted to many panic-like symptoms since the RTA. She also admitted to feeling threatened with death or serious injury.
- She exhibited a re-experiencing of the RTA in the form of recurrent nightmares and flashbacks. She also exhibited symptoms of hyper-arousal in the form of hyper-vigilance and a characteristic startle response.
- There was a long history of PTSD where she had experienced similar anxiety symptoms, which had begun quite specifically after an extreme stress or a life-threatening event, and where she felt similarly threatened with death or serious injury. She had been admitted to hospital with PTSD on three previous occasions, her last admission being some two years earlier following a physical assault when she responded well to **sertraline** 200 mg mane (the maximum dose). She has continued to comply with this medication.
- The working diagnosis is that of a relapse of her PTSD.

What is the psychopharmacological management of this patient?

ANSWER 4

POST-TRAUMATIC STRESS DISORDER (PTSD)

- Selective serotonin reuptake inhibitors (SSRIs) are now considered to be first-line drug treatments in the management of post-traumatic stress disorder (PTSD). The response times to SSRIs are slower in PTSD than in depression.
- The patient has previously responded well, and has been well maintained on the SSRI **sertraline** 200 mg mane (the maximum dose). Unfortunately, however, she has now experienced a relapse of her PTSD despite complying with her medication. There is also no scope for increasing the dosage of the **sertraline** since it is already at the maximum dosage.
- In this instance it is worth considering a switch to a second SSRI before abandoning this class of antidepressant. A good choice for such a second SSRI would be **paroxetine**. Like **sertraline,** this is also licensed for the treatment of PTSD. In fact, **paroxetine** is licensed for this indication in both men and women, in comparison with **sertraline,** which is licensed for this indication in women only. Moreover, **paroxetine** was the first SSRI to have a licence for the treatment of PTSD and it remains the only other SSRI licensed for this indication apart from **sertraline**.
- If the patient fails to respond to the second SSRI **paroxetine,** consider switching to a different class of antidepressant. The noradrenergic and specific serotonergic antidepressant (NaSSA) **mirtazapine*** may be considered as the next antidepressant of choice in the treatment of PTSD, based on a recent review article by Jonathan Bisson.**
- If the patient fails to respond to the NaSSA **mirtazapine**, consider switching to the monoamine-oxidase inhibitor (MAOI) **phenelzine.*** There is evidence of efficacy for its use in PTSD, but it has poor side-effect tolerability.
- If the patient fails to respond to the MAOI **phenelzine**, consider switching to the atypical antipsychotic **olanzapine.***

---

* Used but these indications are not currently licensed in the UK.
** Bisson J. Pharmacological treatment of post traumatic stress disorder. *Advances in Psychiatric Treatment.* 2007; **13**: 119–26.

QUESTION 5

SOCIAL ANXIETY DISORDER

- A 28-year-old Caucasian woman.
- She was assessed in the outpatient clinic by a consultant psychiatrist, after referral by her general practitioner.
- In the outpatient's consultation, she admitted to a fear of, and habit of, avoiding situations in which she may be observed by other people (e.g. restaurants, dinner parties, public transport). She also admitted to a fear that she may behave in a manner that will be humiliating or embarrassing (e.g. blushing, shaking).
- She exhibited anxiety symptoms identical to those of any other anxiety state. She also exhibited anxious thoughts, usually in anticipation of situations she may have to encounter. In addition, she exhibited depersonalisation.
- There was a long history of social anxiety disorder. She was initially referred by her general practitioner to the psychiatric outpatient department 10 years ago with similar anxiety symptoms. Her most recent assessment in the outpatient clinic by a consultant psychiatrist was some six months earlier, when she responded well to **paroxetine** 40 mg mane. She has continued to comply with this medication.
- The working diagnosis is that of a relapse of her social anxiety disorder.

What is the psychopharmacological management of this patient?

ANSWER 5

SOCIAL ANXIETY DISORDER

- Selective serotonin reuptake inhibitors (SSRIs) are now considered to be first-line drug treatments in the management of social anxiety disorder.
- The patient has previously responded well, and has been well maintained on the SSRI **paroxetine** 40 mg mane. Unfortunately, she has experienced a relapse of her social anxiety disorder despite complying with her medication. However, there is scope for increasing the dosage of the **paroxetine** to 50 mg mane (the maximum dose), which may lead to successful clinical remission of the patient's symptoms.
- If the patient fails to respond to **paroxetine** 50 mg mane, it is worth considering a switch to a second SSRI before abandoning this class of antidepressant. A good choice for such a second SSRI would be **escitalopram.** Like **paroxetine,** this is also licensed for the treatment of social anxiety disorder. Moreover, **escitalopram** is the only other SSRI to be licensed for this indication apart from **paroxetine**.
- If the patient fails to respond to the second SSRI **escitalopram,** consider switching to a different class of antidepressant. The reversible inhibitors of monoamine-oxidase type A (RIMAs) may be considered as the next antidepressant class of choice in the treatment of social anxiety disorder, based on standard NICE clinical guidelines and on local trust clinical guidelines. **Moclobemide** (the first RIMA) was introduced into the UK in 1993. It remains the only RIMA available in the UK, and may be considered as a good third-line drug treatment in this patient. Like **paroxetine** and **escitalopram,** it is also licensed for the treatment of social anxiety disorder, cf the monoamine-oxidase inhibitors (MAOIs), which are not licensed for this indication.

QUESTION 6

GENERALISED ANXIETY DISORDER (GAD)

- A 23-year old Caucasian woman.
- Admitted from the psychiatric outpatient clinic by her consultant psychiatrist to the acute unit of the local psychiatric hospital with a six-month history of psychological and physical manifestations of anxiety, not attributable to real danger and occurring as a persisting state.
- She presented at the hospital with the physical symptoms of difficulty in inhaling, the feeling of constriction in her chest, the feeling of discomfort over her heart, excessive wind caused by aerophagy, increased frequency and urgency of micturition, tinnitus and dizziness, aching and stiffness (particularly in the back and shoulders), difficulty getting off to sleep and occasional nightmares (in which she wakes suddenly feeling intensely fearful).
- She exhibited fearful anticipation, irritability, a feeling of restlessness, sensitivity to noise, repetitive worrying thoughts, difficulty in concentration and a subjective report of poor memory.
- This was her first admission to an acute psychiatric unit. She was initially treated by her general practitioner for this episode of illness with the benzodiazepine **diazepam,** which was gradually built up to the maximum dose of 30 mg daily in divided doses (10 mg tds). The **diazepam** helped to reduce her anxiety in the short term. However, because of the risk of drug dependency associated with long-term treatment with benzodiazepines, the **diazepam** was gradually reduced and eventually stopped after four weeks of treatment. Her general practitioner then subsequently started her on the anxiolytic drug **buspirone,** which was gradually built up to the maximum dose of 15 mg tds. Initially, this seemed to help reduce her anxiety, but she subsequently deteriorated despite complying with the **buspirone.** It was this clinical deterioration that resulted in her general practitioner referring her to the psychiatric outpatient clinic.
- The working diagnosis is that of GAD.

What is the psychopharmacological management of this patient?

ANSWER 6

GENERALISED ANXIETY DISORDER (GAD)

- In the first instance it is important to exclude an occult thyroid disorder and caffeinism as a cause of generalised anxiety disorder (GAD).
- Based on standard NICE clinical guidelines and local trust clinical guidelines, a selective serotonin reuptake inhibitor (SSRI) should be used as first-line therapy in the treatment of GAD. In this patient, **paroxetine** could be considered as the SSRI of choice. It was the first SSRI to be given a licence for the treatment of GAD. The dose of **paroxetine** is usually 20 mg mane; this may be increased up to a maximum of 50 mg daily.
- If the patient fails to respond to the SSRI **paroxetine**, consider switching to a second SSRI. In this respect, consider switching to the SSRI **escitalopram**. This has recently been licensed for the treatment of GAD and is currently the only other SSRI apart from **paroxetine** to be licensed for this indication. The dose of **escitalopram** is 10 mg once daily, increased if necessary to a maximum of 20 mg daily.
- If the patient fails to respond to the second SSRI **escitalopram,** consider switching to a different class of antidepressant. The selective noradrenaline reuptake inhibitors (SNRIs) could be considered as the next antidepressant class of choice, based on standard NICE clinical guidelines and local trust clinical guidelines. The SNRI **venlafaxine XL** is currently the only licensed SNRI for GAD. The dose of **venlafaxine XL** is 75 mg daily as a single dose; this should be discontinued if there is no response after eight weeks. Some studies have used 150 mg daily,* although the evidence for greater efficacy is debatable.
- If the patient fails to respond to the SNRI **venlafaxine XL**, consider switching to a different class of antidepressant. The tricyclic and related antidepressant drugs could be considered as the next antidepressant class of choice based on standard NICE clinical guidelines and local trust clinical guidelines. **Trazodone**, an antidepressant drug related to the tricyclic antidepressants (TCAs), may be considered as a good choice in this patient. It is licensed for the treatment of anxiety. The dose of **trazodone** is 75 mg daily, increased if necessary to 300 mg daily. In addition, the TCAs **imipramine** or **dosulepin** could help.
- If the patient fails to respond to a tricyclic and related antidepressant drug, there are some studies that show efficacy with the noradrenergic and specific serotonergic antidepressant (NaSSA) **mirtazapine,**** and this would promote sleep.

* Used but this dosage is not currently licensed in the UK.
** Used but this indication is not currently licensed in the UK.

QUESTION 7

DISSOCIATIVE (CONVERSION) DISORDER

- A 25-year-old Caucasian woman.
- The patient was referred from the Accident and Emergency Department of the local teaching hospital for a psychiatric opinion.
- She presented acutely with hysterical dissociative reactions in the form of psychogenic amnesia (memory impairment), psychogenic fugue (wandering), somnambulism (sleepwalking) and multiple personality (sudden alternations between two patterns of behaviour, each of which is forgotten by the patient when the other is present).
- She also displayed hysterical conversion symptoms in the form of paralysis, fits, blindness and disorders of gait.
- She exhibited primary gain so that anxiety arising from a psychological conflict is excluded from the patient's conscious mind.
- She also exhibited secondary gain so that the hysterical dissociative reactions and the hysterical conversion symptoms she displayed confer some advantage on the patient, for example the attention of others. In addition, she exhibited 'belle indifference', i.e. less than the expected amount of distress often shown by patients with hysterical major dissociative reactions and 'classic' conversion symptoms.
- There are no demonstrable organic disorders; that is, it is important to exclude organic brain disease such as dementia, cerebral tumour, general paralysis of the insane (GPI), multiple sclerosis and complex, partial seizures (temporal lobe epilepsy) before making a diagnosis of dissociative (conversion) disorder.
- In addition, in order to diagnose dissociative (conversion) disorder, it is important to exclude histrionic personality disorder as well as malingering (where the symptoms of illness are deliberately falsified in order to achieve secondary gain).
- Her parents described her as being a happy child until they separated when she was 12 years old. She subsequently coped poorly with puberty and became increasingly histrionic in her behaviour, displaying the characteristic pre-morbid histrionic personality traits of self-dramatisation, a self-centred approach to personal relationships and a craving for excitement and novelty.
- There is a family psychiatric history in that her mother has been diagnosed with a dissociative (conversion) disorder.
- The working diagnosis is that of a first episode of a dissociative (conversion) disorder in the setting of pre-morbid histrionic personality traits.

What is the psychopharmacological management of this patient?

ANSWER 7

DISSOCIATIVE (CONVERSION) DISORDER

- For acute presentations, lasting up to a few weeks (as in this patient), treatment by reassurance and suggestion is usually appropriate and may be sufficient, together with immediate effort to resolve any stressful circumstances which provoked the reaction. In addition, it is important to focus on the elimination of factors that are reinforcing the symptoms, and on the encouragement of normal behaviour.
- However, in view of her past psychosexual history and pre-morbid personality, it is likely that she has deep-seated psychological problems underlying her dissociative (conversion) disorder. In order to address these, psychopharmacological intervention may be required for the purpose of abreaction.
- Classically, abreaction was brought about by an intravenous injection of small amounts of the barbiturate **amylobarbitone sodium.** Nowadays, however, such abreaction can be initiated more safely by a slow intravenous injection of 10 mg of the long-acting benzodiazepine **diazepam**. A male doctor should administer this in the company of a female chaperone to avoid the potential risk of a subsequent complaint owing to false memory/dissociation.
- In the resulting state, the patient is encouraged to re-live the stressful events that provoked the dissociative (conversion) disorder, and to express the accompanying emotions.
- Patients usually respond well to exploratory psychotherapy concerned with their past life. They often produce striking memories of childhood sexual behaviour and other problems apparently relevant to psychodynamic psychotherapy. However, such ideas should not be explored at length since this may lead to over-dependence.

QUESTION 8

PERSISTENT DELUSIONAL DISORDER

- A 31-year-old Asian woman.
- A 10-year history of psychotic illness.
- First episode of psychosis was treated in Pakistan with **haloperidol** 5 mg bd. She made a good recovery from this episode of illness and was subsequently discharged from hospital after two months.
- She later came to the UK and was soon admitted with fairly fixed, elaborate and systematised persecutory delusions in the absence of a primary organic, schizophrenic or affective disorder. She had stopped taking her **haloperidol** one month prior to admission because she experienced extra-pyramidal side-effects (EPSE) on it and suspected that the medication would harm her. A diagnosis of a persistent delusional disorder was made. She responded to **olanzapine** 15 mg nocte, and was subsequently discharged from hospital after two months.
- More recently, she was re-admitted to hospital with a further relapse of her persistent delusional disorder caused by non-compliance with her **olanzapine,** which she stopped taking one month prior to re-admission because she experienced oversedation on it and suspected that the medication would harm her.

What is the psychopharmacological management of this patient?

ANSWER 8

PERSISTENT DELUSIONAL DISORDER

- The patient in this case made a good recovery previously with **olanzapine** 15 mg nocte. Unfortunately, she stopped complying with the medication owing to oversedation. In the first instance, therefore, the patient should be encouraged to restart the **olanzapine,** albeit at the lower dose of 5 mg to 10 mg nocte. The patient should be reassured that the medication should not harm her and that it is hoped that her persistent delusional disorder may be clinically stabilised on this lower dose of **olanzapine** without her experiencing oversedation.
- If the patient continues to experience oversedation on **olanzapine** 5 mg to 10 mg nocte, or if her persistent delusional disorder fails to be clinically stabilised on this lower dose of **olanzapine**, consider switching to the atypical antipsychotic **amisulpride**. This is the least sedative of all the atypical antipsychotic drugs. The usual dose range of **amisulpride** is 200 mg bd to 400 mg bd, with a maximum dosage of 600 mg bd.
- If the patient subsequently develops hyperprolactinaemia associated with clinical manifestations on **amisulpride,** or if her persistent delusional disorder fails to be clinically stabilised on **amisulpride,** consider switching to the atypical antipsychotic **aripiprazole.** This has a prolactin level comparable with placebo, cf **amisulpride.** The usual starting dose of **aripiprazole** is 10 mg to 15 mg once daily with a maximum dose of 30 mg daily.

QUESTION 9

DEPRESSION WITH PANIC ATTACKS

- A 52-year-old Caucasian man.
- He was admitted to hospital with palpitations, pounding heart, tachycardia, sweating, trembling and shortness of breath. He was terrified by this episode and was concerned that he may have suffered with a heart attack.
- On admission, he admitted to sleep disturbance in the form of early morning wakening, loss of appetite, loss of weight and loss of interest in work and pleasure activities for several weeks.
- He exhibited poverty of speech, a depressed mood, anxiety, ideas of hopelessness (the patient expecting the worst), suicidal ideas and poverty of thought.
- There is no past psychiatric history.
- Despite his concerns that he may have suffered with a heart attack, his ECG was entirely normal.
- The working diagnosis is that of a depressive disorder with panic attacks.

What is the psychopharmacological management of this patient?

ANSWER 9

DEPRESSION WITH PANIC ATTACKS

- An antidepressant which is licensed for the treatment of both depressive disorder and panic disorder is indicated in this patient, owing to the panic attacks which accompany the patient's depressive disorder.
- The antidepressant group of choice is a selective serotonin reuptake inhibitor (SSRI), since central serotonin (5-HT) systems have been implicated in the aetiology of both depressive disorder and panic disorder, and thus members of this group of antidepressants are indeed licensed for both depressive disorder and panic disorder. In this patient **citalopram** could be considered as the SSRI of choice, based on standard NICE clinical guidelines and local trust clinical guidelines. **Citalopram** is licensed for the treatment of depressive illness in the initial phase and as maintenance against patient relapse/recurrence of depressive illness. It is also licensed for the treatment of panic disorder with or without agoraphobia.
- If the patient fails to respond to the SSRI **citalopram,** consider switching to a second SSRI. In this respect, consider switching to the SSRI **escitalopram. Escitalopram** is a highly selective SSRI that is effective and well tolerated in the treatment of major depressive episodes and panic disorder with or without agoraphobia. Recent studies have demonstrated differences in efficacy and in the mode of action compared to **citalopram.** There is some evidence that the efficacy of **escitalopram** in the treatment of depression is comparable to the serotonin and noradrenaline reuptake inhibitor (SNRI) **venlafaxine XL,** cf other SSRIs, including **citalopram,** where there is considerable evidence that **venlafaxine XL** is more effective in the treatment of depression. There is also some evidence that **escitalopram** may be associated with an early symptom relief in the treatment of depression, cf **citalopram.** This may be explained by the serotonin transporter theory, which suggests that **escitalopram** functions more effectively than **citalopram** by increasing serotonin levels more than **citalopram.** All of this would suggest that clinically it would make more sense to treat with **escitalopram** ahead of **citalopram.** However, since **citalopram** costs less than **escitalopram,** primary care trusts generally advocate the use of **citalopram** ahead of **escitalopram.**
- If the patient fails to respond to the second SSRI **escitalopram,** consider switching to a different class of antidepressant. The noradrenergic and specific serotonergic antidepressants (NaSSAs) could be considered as the next antidepressant class of choice based on standard NICE clinical guidelines and local trust clinical guidelines. The NaSSA **mirtazapine** may be considered as a good choice in this patient since he is expressing suicidal ideas.

QUESTION 10

NON-RESISTANT DEPRESSION

- A 46-year-old Caucasian male.
- He was admitted to the acute psychiatric unit of his local district general hospital following referral from his general practitioner.
- He presented with a two-month history of weight loss, agitation, feeling depressed, loss of libido, constipation and sleep disturbance in the form of onset insomnia.
- He exhibited morbid thoughts concerned with the past, taking the form of unreasonable guilt and self-blame about minor matters, such as feeling guilty about past trivial acts of dishonesty. In addition, he exhibited a depressed mood, anxiety and suicidal ideas.
- He suffered a severe depressive episode two years ago, which resulted in admission to hospital for a two-month period. His discharge medication was **fluoxetine** 40 mg mane.
- He stopped complying with his medication six months ago and lost contact with psychiatric services.
- Both his mother and father have a diagnosis of depression.
- The working diagnosis is that of a relapse of a non-resistant depressive illness.

What is the psychopharmacological management of this patient?

ANSWER 10

NON-RESISTANT DEPRESSION

- The patient in this case made a good recovery previously with **fluoxetine** 40 mg mane. The reason for his non-compliance with medication is unclear. If adverse effects were not the reason for discontinuing the treatment, the selective serotonin reuptake inhibitor (SSRI) **fluoxetine** should be prescribed again. The best guide to a choice of antidepressant is what worked well in the past; this is mentioned in the NICE guidelines.
- If adverse effects were the reason for discontinuation, an alternative antidepressant with a different side-effect profile should be prescribed.
- If agitation was the adverse effect resulting in discontinuation, consider prescribing the SSRI **citalopram,** which is relatively less alerting owing to its neutral psychomotor profile, cf **fluoxetine,** which is thought to increase psychomotor activity.
- If sexual dysfunction was the adverse effect resulting in discontinuation, consider prescribing the noradrenergic and specific serotonergic antidepressant (NaSSA) **mirtazapine** – the world's first-ever antidepressant available as an orally disintegrating tablet. **Mirtazapine** may lack the serotonin-related side-effect of sexual dysfunction, possibly owing to the blockade of serotonin $5HT_2$ receptors.
- If there are family members who have suffered from depression, the drug that worked well for them may predict a positive response in this patient.

QUESTION 11

RESISTANT DEPRESSION

- A 36-year-old Asian male.
- A 10-year history of depressive illness.
- First episode of depression was treated in Pakistan with **paroxetine** 30 mg mane. He made a good recovery from this episode of illness and was subsequently discharged from hospital after two months.
- He later came to the UK and was soon admitted with feeling depressed, morbid thoughts concerned with the present (with him seeing the unhappy side of every event), poverty of speech, poverty of thought, suicidal thoughts, middle insomnia, appetite loss and weight loss. A diagnosis of depressive disorder was made. He responded to **sertraline** 150 mg mane and was subsequently discharged from hospital after three months.
- More recently, he was re-admitted to hospital with a further relapse of his depressive disorder, which is now resistant to treatment with his previous antidepressant medications.

What is the psychopharmacological management of this patient?

ANSWER 11

RESISTANT DEPRESSION

- Since the patient has proved resistant to treatment with two different selective serotonin reuptake inhibitors (SSRIs), another class of antidepressant drug should now be considered.
- It is worth considering a trial of the serotonin and noradrenaline reuptake inhibitor (SNRI) **duloxetine** – there is some evidence that **duloxetine,** as a member of the SNRI class of antidepressants, is effective in resistant depression.
- If the patient fails to respond to the SNRI **duloxetine**, consider switching to the noradrenergic and specific serotonergic antidepressant (NaSSA) **mirtazapine** – there is some evidence that **mirtazapine,** as a member of the NaSSA class of antidepressants, is effective in resistant depression (**mirtazapine** is indeed in a class of its own, i.e. there are no other antidepressants in the NaSSA class of antidepressants).
- If the patient fails to respond to the NaSSA **mirtazapine,** it is worth considering adding in the SNRI **venlafaxine** to the NaSSA **mirtazapine.** By combining these two different antidepressants, one is effectively treating the resistant depression with two different antidepressant drugs with different modes of action. The combination of **mirtazapine** and high-dose **venlafaxine** is known as 'Californian Rocket Fuel'* – theoretically this is very potent since it boosts the accumulation within the synapse of both serotonin and noradrenaline through a combination of reuptake inhibition, pre-synaptic blockade and post-synaptic blockade.
- If the patient fails to respond to the drug combination of **mirtazapine** and high-dose **venlafaxine,** it is worth considering a course of electroconvulsive therapy (ECT) – the use of ECT for the treatment of resistant depression is well documented and shown to be effective, but it does require the use of a general anaesthetic with the associated risks this carries.
- If the patient fails to respond to ECT, it is worth considering **lithium** augmentation of **mirtazapine** and high-dose **venlafaxine.**

* Used but this indication is not currently licensed in the UK.

QUESTION 12

DEPRESSIVE DISORDER IN A PATIENT WITH EPILEPSY

- A 36-year-old Caucasian woman.
- She was taken by her husband to the Accident and Emergency Department of her local district general hospital.
- She had a 10-year history of resistant temporal lobe epilepsy (complex partial seizures).
- Presented with feeling depressed, amenorrhoea, constipation, agitation, loss of libido, initial insomnia and morbid thoughts concerned with the future accompanied by the thoughts that life is no longer worth living and that death would come as a welcome release.
- She exhibited a depressed mood, suicidal thoughts and poverty of speech.
- She was subsequently admitted to the local psychiatric unit.
- Two months prior to admission, her general practitioner had diagnosed her with a depressive disorder and prescribed **dosulepin** 150 mg nocte, which she had complied with. Her anti-epileptic on admission was **sodium valproate** 1.2 grams bd and **carbamazepine** 200 mg bd.
- Following admission she was observed to have daily epileptic seizures (one a day) for the first week.
- The advice of a consultant neurologist was sought, and, as a result, her **carbamazepine** was gradually increased to 400 mg bd. Her epileptic seizures subsequently stopped. The patient continued to display depressive symptoms.
- The working diagnosis was that of an inter-ictal depressive disorder, that is, a depressive disorder occurring independently of epileptic seizures.

What is the psychopharmacological management of this patient?

ANSWER 12

DEPRESSIVE DISORDER IN A PATIENT WITH EPILEPSY

- In inter-ictal depressive disorder, to prevent relapse it is necessary to continue antidepressant medication for six months following clinical recovery after the first episode of the disorder, and for several (one to three) years following clinical recovery after two or more episodes of the disorder.
- When choosing an antidepressant drug in a patient with epilepsy, it is important to take into account what effects the antidepressant has on lowering the seizure threshold, and whether the antidepressant is likely to interact with any anti-epileptic medication the patient is taking.
- In this patient, consider switching to an antidepressant with a low pro-convulsive effect, since **dosulepin** is one of the most epileptogenic of the older tricyclic antidepressant drugs (TCAs).
- The reversible inhibitor of monoamine oxidase type A (RIMA) **moclo-bemide** may be the antidepressant of choice in this patient. It is not known to be pro-convulsive. In addition, there are no known clinically significant interactions with the anti-convulsants **carbamazepine** and **sodium valproate**.
- If the patient fails to respond to the RIMA **moclobemide,** consider switching to the selective serotonin reuptake inhibitor (SSRI) **citalo-pram.** It has a low pro-convulsive effect. However, **carbamazepine** may increase its rate of metabolism and larger doses of **citalopram** may be required. Seizure risk is dose-related. **Citalopram** may be the safest SSRI to use in epilepsy, but seizures have been reported in overdose.
- If the patient fails to respond to the SSRI **citalopram**, consider switching to **trazodone** – an antidepressant drug related to the TCAs, but a more selective inhibitor of the reuptake of serotonin, cf **amitriptyline** and **imipramine. Trazodone** has a low pro-convulsive effect. However, **carbamazepine** increases its rate of metabolism and **sodium valproate** decreases its rate of metabolism. Seizure risk is dose-related.
- It is worth considering measuring anti-convulsant levels, if only to check compliance.

QUESTION 13

DEPRESSIVE DISORDER IN A PATIENT WITH CARDIOVASCULAR DISEASE

- A 61-year-old Caucasian man.
- He had a 10-year history of hypertension.
- He suffered with a myocardial infarction (MI) three months ago, for which he was treated and subsequently discharged from a general medical ward of his local district general hospital.
- In the past 10 years he has been treated three times for a depressive disorder, each time with **amitriptyline** 150 mg nocte.
- Presented with a two-month history of feeling depressed, excessive sleeping but still feeling unrefreshed on waking, loss of appetite, loss of energy and loss of motivation.
- He exhibited a depressed mood and hesitancy of speech, i.e. a long delay before questions were answered.
- His partner was concerned about him and made an appointment for him to see his local general practitioner, who subsequently referred him to his local community mental health team (CMHT).
- His current medication at the time of the referral from his general practitioner was **aspirin** 75 mg od, **atenolol** 50 mg od, **simvastatin** 20 mg od and **enalapril** 20 mg od.
- The working diagnosis is that of a relapse of a depressive disorder occurring post-MI.

What is the psychopharmacological management of this patient?

ANSWER 13

DEPRESSIVE DISORDER IN A PATIENT WITH CARDIOVASCULAR DISEASE

- When choosing an antidepressant drug in a patient with a depressive disorder occurring post-myocardial infarction (post-MI), it is important to consider cardiotoxicity and also the potential for drug interactions with other prescribed medications.
- In this patient, consider switching to an antidepressant with a benign cardiovascular profile since **amitriptyline**, being one of the tricyclic antidepressants (TCAs), is contraindicated in such a patient with a recent MI because of its adverse cardiovascular profile.
- The selective serotonin reuptake inhibitors (SSRIs) appear to have a benign cardiovascular profile and may be considered the antidepressant class of choice in a patient with cardiovascular disease.
- The SSRI **sertraline** may be the antidepressant of choice in this patient. There are no licence restrictions post-MI. It is considered safe post-MI. It is the only antidepressant which has so far been studied in the treatment of depression in post-MI patients (study published in 1999). It may also have a lower potential for drug interactions – since it has no significant interaction with cytochrome P450 2D6.
- If the patient fails to respond to the SSRI **sertraline**, consider switching to a second SSRI. In this respect, consider switching to the SSRI **citalopram**. This should be used with caution – it has a minor metabolite, which may increase the QT_c interval. It is important to keep this interval well below 500 ms. However, it may have a lower potential for drug interactions since it has no significant interaction with cytochrome P450 2D6.
- If the patient fails to respond to the second SSRI **citalopram**, consider switching to a different class of antidepressant. The noradrenergic and specific serotonergic antidepressant (NaSSA) **mirtazapine** may be considered as a good third-line choice for this patient. It is thought to lack cardiovascular side-effects owing to a very low affinity for alpha-1 (α_1) adrenergic receptors. However, it should be used with caution and clinical experience is limited. It is important to watch for weight gain, a common side-effect of **mirtazapine**, and a serious problem in a patient with existing heart disease.

QUESTION 14

RETARDED DEPRESSION

- A 42-year-old Caucasian woman.
- She was referred by her general practitioner to the Outpatient Department.
- She presented with a two-month history of feeling depressed, with excessive sleep but still feeling unrefreshed on waking. In addition, she presented with increased appetite, increased weight, psychomotor retardation, diurnal variation in mood with her feeling worse in the evening, loss of interest in work and pleasure activities, loss of energy, and fatigue, loss of libido, constipation and amenorrhoea.
- She exhibited neglected dress and grooming but maintained a smiling exterior while depressed. She also exhibited poverty of speech, hesitancy of speech with a long delay before questions were answered, a depressed mood qualitatively different from normal unhappiness, loss of reactivity of her mood to circumstances, morbid thoughts concerned with the past in the form of feeling guilty about past trivial acts of dishonesty and poverty of thought.
- For the last month she has been treated by her general practitioner with the selective serotonin reuptake inhibitor (SSRI) **fluoxetine,** at a dose of 20 mg mane, with little improvement.
- There is no past psychiatric history.
- There is a family psychiatric history in that both her father and her brother have been diagnosed with depressive disorders.
- The working diagnosis is that of a first episode of retarded depression (i.e. a depressive disorder with psychomotor retardation as the dominant feature).

What is the psychopharmacological management of this patient?

ANSWER 14

RETARDED DEPRESSION

- In view of the retarded nature of her depression, the patient should be treated with an alerting antidepressant (i.e. one that increase psychomotor activity).
- The drug of choice in retarded depression may be considered to be **fluoxetine** – the most alerting SSRI. Her general practitioner has already initiated her on this medication at the lowest effective dose of 20 mg mane. Although she has shown little improvement on this medication after one month, it is worth increasing the dosage of this medication to see if she responds – it may be increased up to a maximum of 80 mg mane by gradual 20 mg increments, if necessary.
- If the patient fails to respond to the SSRI **fluoxetine,** consider switching to the noradrenaline reuptake inhibitor (NARI) **reboxetine.** This is a highly selective noradrenaline reuptake inhibitor, and thus may be considered a useful drug in the treatment of a depressive disorder with psychomotor retardation as the dominant feature. The starting dose of **reboxetine** is 4 mg bd – if further clinical improvement is required this may be increased to 6 mg mane, 4 mg nocte and, again if necessary, to the maximum dose of 6 mg bd.
- If the patient fails to respond to the NARI **reboxetine,** consider switching to the second-generation antidepressant **lofepramine.** This acts mainly as a noradrenergic reuptake inhibitor, that is, it is a relatively selective reuptake inhibitor of noradrenaline. In view of its alerting nature, it may be considered a useful drug in the treatment of retarded depression. The starting dose of **lofepramine** is 140 mg daily in divided doses – if further clinical improvement is required, this may be increased up to the maximum dosage of 210 mg daily in divided doses.
- If the patient fails to respond to the second-generation antidepressant **lofepramine,** consider admitting her to hospital for a course of electroconvulsive therapy (ECT). The effects of ECT are best in severe depressive disorders, in particular those marked by biological features of depression. She has presented with characteristic psychomotor retardation (i.e. a change in her psychomotor activity so that she is slowed up), which is a good clinical indicator that she may respond to a course of ECT.
- If the patient fails to respond to ECT, it is worth considering **lithium** augmentation of **lofepramine.**
- If the patient fails to respond to the combination of **lithium** and **lofepramine,** consider switching to a monoamine oxidase inhibitor (MAOI) – there are some studies which advise that MAOIs can have an alerting effect in retarded depression.

QUESTION 15

PSYCHOTIC DEPRESSION

- A 48-year-old Caucasian man.
- He was referred from the Accident and Emergency Department of the local district general hospital for a psychiatric opinion.
- He presented with a one-month history of feeling depressed, with early morning wakening, loss of appetite, loss of weight and suicidal ideas. In addition, he presented with the delusional belief that he had cancer and the delusional belief that other people were about to take revenge on him, accepting the supposed persecution as something he had brought upon himself.
- He exhibited a depressed mood with reduced rate of blinking and reduced gestural movements with an appearance of shoulders bent, head inclined forwards and direction of gaze downwards. In addition, he exhibited hypochondriacal delusions (i.e. delusions of ill-health), persecutory delusions and second-person auditory hallucinations in the form of voices addressing repetitive phrases to the patient. The voices confirmed the patient's ideas of worthlessness, for example 'You are an evil man; you should die'. He also exhibited visual hallucinations in the form of scenes of death and destruction.
- He has failed to respond to **dosulepin** (formerly known as **dothiepin**), 150 mg nocte for six weeks, initiated by his general practitioner.
- There is no past psychiatric history.
- There is a family psychiatric history in that both his mother and sister have been diagnosed with depressive disorders.
- The working diagnosis is that of a first episode of psychotic depression (i.e. a depressive disorder with psychotic features).

What is the psychopharmacological management of this patient?

ANSWER 15

PSYCHOTIC DEPRESSION

- In view of the patient's suicidal ideas, consider switching to another antidepressant drug – if taken in overdosage, **dosulepin** is the tricyclic antidepressant (TCA) most commonly responsible for deaths in the UK at present.
- Prefer to switch to one of the selective serotonin reuptake inhibitors (SSRIs), which are safer in overdosage than the TCAs. From among the SSRIs, **citalopram** may be considered as a good choice in the first instance.
- If the patient fails to respond to **citalopram** after an adequate trial, consider switching to a different class of antidepressant for someone this ill. A good choice would be the serotonin and noradrenaline reuptake inhibitors (SNRIs). From among the SNRIs, **duloxetine** may be considered as a good choice.
- In view of the hypochondriacal delusions, persecutory delusions, second-person auditory hallucinations and visual hallucinations, consider adding in an atypical antipsychotic drug to the SNRI. From among the atypical antipsychotics, **olanzapine** may be considered as a good choice in the first instance, and may help promote sleep.
- If the patient fails to respond to **olanzapine** after an adequate trial, consider switching to another antipsychotic drug. The typical antipsychotic **haloperidol** may be considered as a good choice as a second-line antipsychotic.
- If the patient fails to respond to the combination of an SNRI and an antipsychotic drug, consider a course of electroconvulsive therapy (ECT).

QUESTION 16

NON-RESISTANT BIPOLAR AFFECTIVE DISORDER (MANIA)

- A 46-year-old Caucasian lady.
- She was admitted to the acute psychiatric unit of the local district general hospital, after being detained by the police under Section 136 of the Mental Health Act 1983, having been found wandering the streets in the early hours of the morning dressed in her night attire.
- She presented with the belief that she was a religious prophet and also the belief that other people were conspiring against her because of her special importance. In addition, she was verbally aggressive.
- She exhibited expansive ideas, believing that her ideas were original, that her opinions were important and that her work was of outstanding quality. She also exhibited flight of ideas with her thoughts and conversation moving quickly from one topic to another, so that one train of thought was not completed before another appeared.
- She had suffered with two previous episodes of bipolar affective disorder (mania) within the last five years. Both episodes resulted in admission to hospital for a two-month period. Her most recent admission was two years ago when her discharge medication was **lithium carbonate** 800 mg nocte.
- She stopped complying with her medication two months ago and lost contact with psychiatric services.
- Both her mother and father have a diagnosis of bipolar affective disorder.
- The working diagnosis is that of a relapse of bipolar affective disorder (mania).

What is the psychopharmacological management of this patient?

ANSWER 16

NON-RESISTANT BIPOLAR AFFECTIVE DISORDER (MANIA)

- The patient in this case made a good recovery previously with the antimanic drug **lithium carbonate** 800 mg nocte. The reason for her non-compliance with medication is unclear. If adverse effects were not the reason for discontinuing treatment, **lithium carbonate** should be prescribed again. The plasma lithium level should be checked – if it is below 0.8 mmol/l, the dosage of **lithium carbonate** should be increased to produce a maximum plasma level of 1.0 mmol/l of lithium.
- If adverse effects were the reason for discontinuation, an alternate antimanic drug with a different side-effect profile should be prescribed. **Valproate semisodium** may be considered as a suitable first-line alternative antimanic drug.
- If the response to an antimanic drug alone is not adequate, consider adding in an antipsychotic drug. Moreover, since this patient's mania presents with psychotic symptoms, there is also a case for initial treatment to include an antipsychotic drug alongside the antimanic drug.
- Historically, **haloperidol** has been the antipsychotic drug of choice in mania. However, in recent years the atypical antipsychotic drug **olanzapine** has been licensed for both the acute phase and for the prophylaxis of mania, and it may now be considered to be the antipsychotic drug of choice in mania.
- If the response to the antimanic drug and the antipsychotic drug remains inadequate at the beginning of treatment, consider adding a short-term benzodiazepine such as **lorazepam** for behavioural disturbance or agitation.
- As this is the patient's third episode of mania within five years, consideration should be given for continuing the antimanic drug* for three years (if not longer) for prophylaxis. The benzodiazepine should be gradually reduced and stopped over a maximum period of four weeks prior to discharge from hospital. Consider cautiously reducing and eventually stopping the antipsychotic drug as an outpatient if possible; however, it may be that she will need to continue on this medication for prophylactic purposes alongside the antimanic drug to prevent a relapse of her mania.

* Valproate semisodium is used but this indication is not currently licensed in the UK.

QUESTION 17

RESISTANT BIPOLAR AFFECTIVE DISORDER (MANIA)

- A 41-year-old Caucasian man.
- He was admitted to the acute psychiatric unit of the local district general hospital, having been detained by the police under Section 136 of the Mental Health Act 1983, having been found wandering in the middle of a busy main road trying to stop traffic.
- He presented with the belief that he was the Messiah. He admitted to hearing the voice of God talking to him and telling him that he had special powers. He also said that he was able to see God.
- He exhibited an elated mood, pressure of speech and flight of ideas. He also exhibited grandiose delusions, second-person auditory hallucinations and visual hallucinations with a religious content. Cognitively, he had impaired attention and concentration, being easily drawn to irrelevancies.
- He had suffered with two previous episodes of bipolar affective disorder (mania) over the last six years. Each episode resulted in admission to hospital for a three-month period. He was discharged on **lithium carbonate** (as **Priadel**) 1.2 grams nocte, associated with a plasma lithium level of 1.0 mmol/l after the first admission. His most recent admission was three years ago when his discharge medication was **valproate semisodium** 1 gram bd. He has complied with both of these medications. However, he is now resistant to treatment with his previous antimanic drugs.
- The working diagnosis is that of a relapse of a bipolar affective disorder (mania).

What is the psychopharmacological management of this patient?

ANSWER 17

RESISTANT BIPOLAR AFFECTIVE DISORDER (MANIA)

- In the first instance, consideration needs to be given to the treatment of the acute episode of bipolar affective disorder (mania) – consider using the atypical antipsychotic **olanzapine** as a first-line agent to this end. This can be added into **valproate semisodium** 1 gram bd. The starting dose of **olanzapine** is 10 mg nocte when used for the treatment of acute mania in combination with an antimanic drug. It may be built up to a maximum dose of 20 mg nocte, if required.
- Once the patient has recovered from the acute episode of mania, consideration needs to be given to the prophylaxis of bipolar affective disorder (mania) – consider continuing the **valproate semisodium*** and **olanzapine** in combination to this end, since the patient is already on the maximum dose of **valproate semisodium** 1 gram bd and has broken down on this medication when taken as monotherapy, although he did remain stable and out of hospital while taking it for nearly three years.
- If the patient has subsequent frequent relapses or continuing functional impairment on **valproate semisodium** and **olanzapine**, consider adding in **lithium carbonate** to the drug regimen. The patient has previously remained stable and out of hospital on **lithium carbonate** while taking it for nearly three years, albeit he did break down on this medication when taking it as monotherapy at the maximum dose of 1.2 gram nocte (which was associated with a plasma level of 1.0 mmol/l). The triple combination of **valproate semisodium, olanzapine** and **lithium carbonate** is regarded as a robust drug regimen for the prophylaxis of bipolar affective disorder (mania).
- If this triple combination of **valproate semisodium, olanzapine** and **lithium carbonate** proves ineffective for prophylaxis, consider substituting **carbamazepine** for **valproate semisodium,** that is, consider the triple combination of **carbamazepine, lithium carbonate** and **olanzapine** for subsequent prophylaxis of bipolar affective disorder (mania). **Carbamazepine** and **lithium carbonate** appear to have a synergistic effect when used in combination. However, the concurrent use of **carbamazepine** with **lithium carbonate** may result in neurotoxicity without raising the plasma lithium level; hence, if **carbamazepine** is added to **lithium carbonate** it should be done so with caution, cf the concurrent use of **valproate semisodium** with **lithium carbonate,** which is safe.
- If this triple combination of **carbamazepine, lithium carbonate** and **olanzapine** proves neurotoxic, consider substituting **lamotrigine*** for **carbamazepine;** that is, consider the triple combination of **lamotrigine, lithium carbonate** and **olanzapine** for subsequent prophylaxis of bipolar affective disorder (mania).

* Used but these indications are not currently licensed in the UK.

QUESTION 18

RAPID-CYCLING BIPOLAR AFFECTIVE DISORDER

- A 30-year-old Caucasian woman.
- She was taken by her husband to the Accident and Emergency Department of her local district general hospital.
- She had a 10-year history of bipolar affective disorder, including four affective episodes within the last 12 months.
- She was subsequently admitted to the local psychiatric unit where she has remained as an inpatient for the last four months.
- She has not been observed to be euthymic in mood throughout this period of time. Her mood has changed rapidly from one of euphoria with infectious gaiety to one of misery with a loss of reactivity to circumstances. Each mood state lasts only for a few days. When feeling depressed, she has morbid thoughts concerned with the future – these take the form of ideas of hopelessness with the patient expecting the worst. In addition, on one occasion these morbid thoughts have progressed to thoughts of, and plans for, suicide.
- Her current medication is **lithium carbonate** (as **Priadel**) 1.2 gram nocte and **sertraline** 150 mg mane. Her plasma lithium level is 1.0 mmol/l.
- The working diagnosis is that of a rapid-cycling bipolar affective disorder (four or more affective episodes per year).

What is the psychopharmacological management of this patient?

ANSWER 18

RAPID-CYCLING BIPOLAR AFFECTIVE DISORDER

- In the first instance, in order to optimise her psychopharmacological treatment the antidepressant should be withdrawn, that is, the logical first step is the withdrawal of the **sertraline.**
- If she continues to rapid-cycle once the **sertraline** has been withdrawn, her ongoing management with **lithium carbonate (Priadel)** needs to be addressed.
- Her plasma lithium level is already at the maximum of 1.0 mmol/l, which does not allow any scope for increasing the dose of **lithium carbonate (Priadel)** above 1.2 gram nocte. This would classify her as a rapid-cycling lithium non-responder.
- Thus, as a rapid-cycling lithium non-responder, consideration would then need to be given to switching her to an alternative antimanic drug that is also licensed for rapid-cycling bipolar affective disorder. The logical drug of choice would be **carbamazepine**. This is licensed for the prophylaxis of bipolar affective disorder in patients who are unresponsive to **lithium.** Moreover, it seems to be particularly effective in patients with rapid-cycling bipolar affective disorder.
- If switching to **carbamazepine** is ineffective, consider reintroducing **lithium carbonate (Priadel)** and using the combination of **lithium carbonate** and **carbamazepine** to stabilise her rapid-cycling bipolar affective disorder – this combination is sometimes effective in patients where the individual drugs used as monotherapy have proved ineffective.
- The following points are also worth mentioning:
  (a) The need to ensure good suppression of thyroid stimulating hormone (TSH).
  (b) **Lamotrigine*** can be useful.
  (c) According to Maudsley guidelines, the following agents may also be useful:
     Quetiapine.*
     Risperidone.*
     Clozapine.*
     Nimodipine.*

*Used but these indications are not currently licensed in the UK.

QUESTION 19

ANTIDEPRESSANT-INDUCED SWITCHING TO MANIA IN BIPOLAR AFFECTIVE DISORDER

- A 31-year-old Caucasian woman.
- Admitted to the acute psychiatric unit of the local district general hospital, having been detained by the police under Section 136 of the Mental Health Act 1983, after they had been called out to a local cinema where she was reported to be running up and down the aisles shouting and screaming in a disinhibited manner.
- She presented at the hospital with the belief that she was a religious prophet and the belief that a remark heard on television was directed specifically to her (i.e. had a personal significance for her).
- She exhibited an elated mood, pressure of speech, pressure of thought and flight of ideas. She also exhibited grandiose delusions and delusions of reference. She was untidy and dishevelled in her appearance. With regard to her clothing, she was wearing bright colours and had an ill-assorted choice of garments.
- She had suffered with five previous episodes of bipolar affective disorder over the last 10 years. Her first admission, 10 years ago, for mania responded to antipsychotic medication. Following her second admission, eight years ago, for mania, she was discharged on **lithium carbonate (Priadel)** 800 mg nocte. She remained stable on this medication for the first three years, but then began to suffer from major depressive episodes. Over the last five years she has had three psychiatric admissions: two of these admissions have been for major depressive disorders, whilst one of the admissions was for mania, which occurred two months after initiating treatment with the antidepressant **lofepramine.** During her last admission for a major depressive episode, three months ago, she was started on the antidepressant **venlafaxine XL** 75 mg daily, the dose of which has cautiously been increased over the last two months to 150 mg daily. She has been prescribed this dose of **venlafaxine XL** for one month prior to her current admission to hospital.
- Both her mother and father have a diagnosis of bipolar affective disorder.
- Her current medication is **lithium carbonate (Priadel)** 1.2 gram nocte and **venlafaxine XL** 150 mg daily.
- Her plasma lithium level is 1.0 mmol/l.
- The working diagnosis is that of an antidepressant-induced switching to mania in bipolar affective disorder.

What is the psychopharmacological management of this patient?

ANSWER 19

ANTIDEPRESSANT-INDUCED SWITCHING TO MANIA IN BIPOLAR AFFECTIVE DISORDER

- Antidepressant-induced switching is defined as the induction by antidepressants of mania or hypomania in patients with bipolar affective disorder or unipolar affective disorder (unipolar depression). It can also be defined as the induction by antidepressants of an increase in the rate of cycling.
- In the first instance, in order to optimise her psychopharmacological treatment, the antidepressant should be stopped abruptly, that is, the logical first step is abruptly to stop the **venlafaxine XL**.
- If she continues to display clinical features of antidepressant-induced switching to mania once the **venlafaxine XL** has been stopped abruptly, her ongoing management with **lithium carbonate (Priadel)** needs to be addressed. Her plasma lithium level is already at the maximum of 1.0 mmol/l, which does not allow any scope for increasing the dose of **lithium carbonate (Priadel)** above 1.2 gram nocte. This would classify her as a lithium non-responder.
- As a lithium non-responder, consideration would then need to be given to switching her to an alternative antimanic drug. Based on standard NICE clinical guidelines and on local trust clinical guidelines, consider switching the patient from **lithium carbonate (Priadel)** to **valproate semisodium**.
- Ideally, such a patient with bipolar affective disorder should be managed in the long term with an antimanic drug alone; that is, **valproate semisodium*** should be used as monotherapy for prophylaxis. However, if the patient were to suffer with another major depressive episode, consideration would need to be given to adding in an antidepressant to the antimanic drug. The class of antidepressants that may be considered to be least likely to induce switching to mania in bipolar affective disorder is the selective serotonin reuptake inhibitors (SSRIs). From the SSRIs, **citalopram** may be considered as the drug of choice for use in this patient.

* Used but this indication is not currently licensed in the UK.

QUESTION 20

BIPOLAR AFFECTIVE DISORDER (DEPRESSION) – BIPOLAR DEPRESSION

- A 31-year-old Caucasian woman.
- She was admitted to hospital by her consultant psychiatrist from the psychiatric outpatient clinic, having been accompanied there by her husband.
- She presented with early morning wakening (middle insomnia) occurring two to three hours before her usual time. She said that she did not fall asleep, but lay awake, feeling unrefreshed, with depressive thinking. She also presented with loss of energy and fatigue.
- She exhibited morbid thoughts concerned with the present, with her no longer feeling confident and discounting any success as a chance happening, for which she could take no credit. Her mood was one of misery, which was qualitatively different from normal unhappiness. She also exhibited poverty of thought and suicidal thoughts.
- She was first admitted to hospital with an episode of bipolar affective disorder (mania) six years ago. She was discharged on **lithium carbonate (Priadel)** 800 mg nocte. Four years ago she was re-admitted to hospital with her first episode of bipolar affective disorder (depression). She was discharged on **lithium carbonate (Priadel)** 1 gram nocte and **citalopram** 20 mg daily. Two years ago she was again re-admitted to hospital with bipolar affective disorder (depression). Following a lengthy admission, she was discharged on **lithium carbonate (Priadel)** 1.2 gram nocte, associated with a plasma lithium level of 1.0 mmol/l, and **citalopram** 40 mg daily. She has complied with both of these medications subsequently.
- The working diagnosis is that of a relapse of a bipolar affective disorder (depression).

What is the psychopharmacological management of this patient?

ANSWER 20

BIPOLAR AFFECTIVE DISORDER (DEPRESSION) – BIPOLAR DEPRESSION

- In the first instance, consideration needs to be given to the treatment of the acute episode of bipolar affective disorder (depression) – consider increasing the dose of the antidepressant **citalopram** to the maximum of 60 mg daily.
- Once the patient has recovered from the acute episode of depression, consideration needs to be given to the prophylaxis of bipolar affective disorder (depression) – consider continuing **lithium carbonate (Priadel)** 1.2 gram nocte and **citalopram** 60 mg daily in combination, to this end.
- If the patient has subsequent frequent relapses or continuing functional impairment on **lithium carbonate (Priadel)** and **citalopram**, consider switching the patient to **lamotrigine*** – this appears to be effective in the prophylaxis of bipolar depression and it does not induce rapid cycling or switching in bipolar affective disorder.
- If switching to **lamotrigine** is ineffective, consider further switching the patient to the combination of **olanzapine** and **fluoxetine** ('zyp–zac')* – this combination appears to be effective in the prophylaxis of bipolar depression.

* Used but these indications are not currently licensed in the UK.

QUESTION 21

BIPOLAR AFFECTIVE DISORDER (ACUTE MANIA) IN PREGNANCY

- A 32-year-old Caucasian woman.
- She was admitted to hospital owing to a deteriorating mental state.
- She presented with a three-week history of reduced sleep, but no fatigue, with the patient waking early, feeling lively and energetic, often getting up and busying herself noisily to the surprise of other people. She had increased appetite, with food eaten greedily with little attention to conventional manners. She also had weight loss attributed to over-activity. In addition, she had increased energy without fatigue and increased libido with uninhibited behaviour, which led to her neglecting precautions against pregnancy.
- She was untidy and dishevelled in her appearance and she wore clothing with bright colours with an ill-assorted choice of garments. She exhibited pressure of speech, pressure of thought, flight of ideas, and her mood was one of euphoria with infectious gaiety.
- She had been diagnosed with bipolar affective disorder (mania) 10 years ago, on her first hospital admission. She has had two subsequent manic relapses, both of which were precipitated by non-compliance with oral antimanic medication (**lithium carbonate** the first time, **carbamazepine** the second time) as a result of adverse effects. During her last admission four years ago, she was prescribed the antimanic drug **valproate semisodium** 750 mg bd, on which she remained clinically stable up to her recent deterioration. She has remained compliant with her antimanic medication for the last four years.
- The working diagnosis is that of a relapse of a bipolar affective disorder (acute mania).
- Following this admission to hospital a pregnancy test was done, which was positive. A subsequent ultrasound scan confirmed that she was approximately two months pregnant.

What is the psychopharmacological management of this patient?

ANSWER 21

BIPOLAR AFFECTIVE DISORDER (ACUTE MANIA) IN PREGNANCY

- **Valproate semisodium** should not be routinely prescribed in the treatment of bipolar affective disorder (acute mania) in pregnancy owing to its having a clear causal link with an increased risk of a variety of foetal abnormalities, in particular spina bifida. This teratogenic effect is probably dose-related. If possible, **valproate semisodium** is probably best avoided in pregnancy.
- In this patient, consider switching to an oral conventional anti-psychotic drug due to their safety data and because there is more clinical experience with them, cf oral atypical antipsychotic drugs.
- The conventional antipsychotic drug **haloperidol** would be a good choice in this patient. There has been widespread use of **haloperidol** in pregnancy and it is recommended by some clinicians as the anti-psychotic of choice.
- If the patient fails to respond to **haloperidol,** consider switching to the atypical antipsychotic **olanzapine.** It is licensed as monotherapy for both the treatment of acute mania as well as for the prophylaxis of bipolar affective disorder. In addition, it is one of the atypical anti-psychotics with the most data, and it is widely used by perinatal services in the UK.
- If the patient fails to respond to **olanzapine,** and the mania is severe, consider a course of electroconvulsive therapy (ECT).
- If there is no alternative to using **valproate semisodium,** use the lowest possible dose due to its probable dose-related teratogenic effect. In addition, the patient should take **folic acid** (5 mg daily), which may reduce the risk of neonatal neural tube defects. The teratogenic effect may be monitored with foetal ultrasound scans, and early intervention with pregnancy termination may be an option.

QUESTION 22

NON-RESISTANT SCHIZOPHRENIA

- A 26-year-old Caucasian man.
- He was taken to the police station by the police under Section 136 of the Mental Health Act 1983.
- He presented with a two-month history of thought broadcasting, hallucinatory voices giving a running commentary on his behaviour and the persistent delusion of being in communication with aliens.
- He exhibited loosening of associations with knight's move thinking (derailment) and incongruity of affect.
- He suffered with a psychotic episode two years ago, which resulted in admission to hospital for a two-month period. His discharge medication was **flupenthixol decanoate** depot injection 40 mg once every two weeks and **procyclidine** 5 mg bd.
- He stopped complying with his medication six months ago and lost contact with psychiatric services.
- Both his mother and father have a diagnosis of schizophrenia.
- The working diagnosis is that of a relapse of a non-resistant schizophrenic illness.

What is the psychopharmacological management of this patient?

ANSWER 22

NON-RESISTANT SCHIZOPHRENIA

- The patient in this case made a good recovery previously with **flupenthixol decanoate** depot injection 40 mg once every two weeks. The reason for his non-compliance with medication is unclear. If adverse effects were not the reason for discontinuing treatment, **flupenthixol decanoate** depot injection should be prescribed again.
- If adverse effects were the reason for discontinuation, an alternative antipsychotic depot injection with a different side-effect profile should be prescribed.
- If agitation was the adverse effect resulting in discontinuation, consider prescribing the depot injection **zuclopenthixol decanoate** in view of its sedative nature; cf **flupenthixol decanoate,** which is considered to be alerting in nature and thus can cause over-excitement.
- If extra pyramidal side-effects (EPSEs) were the adverse effects resulting in discontinuation, consider prescribing intramuscular (IM) **risperidone** – the world's first-ever atypical antipsychotic long-acting intramuscular injection. IM **risperidone** is considered to have fewer EPSEs, cf conventional antipsychotic depot injections.

QUESTION 23

RESISTANT SCHIZOPHRENIA

- A 34-year-old Asian man.
- A 10-year history of psychotic illness.
- First episode of psychosis was treated in Pakistan with **haloperidol** 5 mg tds. He made a good recovery from this episode of illness and was subsequently discharged from hospital after two months.
- He later came to the UK and was soon admitted with persecutory delusions, third-person auditory hallucinations, 'made' volition and word salad (verbigeration). A diagnosis of schizophrenia was made. He responded to **risperidone** 6 mg mane, and was subsequently discharged from hospital after three months.
- More recently, he was re-admitted to hospital with a further relapse of his schizophrenia, which is now resistant to treatment with his previous antipsychotic medications.

What is the psychopharmacological management of this patient?

ANSWER 23

RESISTANT SCHIZOPHRENIA

- As the patient is now resistant to treatment with his two previous antipsychotic medications (including one atypical), based on standard NICE clinical guidelines and local trust clinical guidelines, it is worth considering a trial of **clozapine** – this is the only drug shown unequivocally to be effective in resistant schizophrenia. Unfortunately, it causes agranulocytosis (life-threatening) in 2% to 3% of patients taking the drug. Its use is therefore restricted to patients registered with the Clozaril Patient Monitoring Service (CPMS), whereby the patient has regular full blood counts to detect any possible agranulocytosis; should this occur, the **clozapine** must be stopped.
- If the patient partially responds to **clozapine** 900 mg daily (maximum dose), it would be worth considering the addition of the atypical antipsychotic **amisulpride** – there is some evidence that the combination of **clozapine** and **amisulpride** is effective in resistant schizophrenia. By combining the serotonin dopamine antagonist (SDA) **clozapine** with the limbic selective dopamine D_3 receptor and D_2 receptor blocker **amisulpride,** one is effectively treating the resistant schizophrenia with two atypical drugs with different modes of action. It would be recommended to do regular ECG monitoring with such a drug regimen (particularly in the early stages of treatment) owing to the theoretical increased risk of prolongation of the QT_c interval. Periodic monitoring of electrolytes is also recommended.
- If the patient fails to fully respond to the combination of **clozapine** 900 mg daily (maximum dose) and **amisulpride** 600 mg bd (maximum dose), based on the Royal College of Psychiatrists' clinical guidelines it is worth considering a course of electroconvulsive therapy (ECT) – there is some evidence that ECT is effective in resistant schizophrenia, although its benefits are only really in the short term.

QUESTION 24

SCHIZOPHRENIA WITH NEGATIVE SYMPTOMS

- A 24-year-old Caucasian man.
- He was living in supported accommodation.
- Visited at home and monitored in the community by his community psychiatric nurse (CPN), who also administers his depot antipsychotic injection of **zuclopenthixol decanoate** 300 mg once every two weeks. In addition, the patient takes **procyclidine** 5 mg tds.
- Staff at the supported accommodation have reported that he has had increasing problems recently, with apathy, lack of drive and initiative, social withdrawal, blunting of affect, poverty of thought, deterioration in his self-care and thought echo.
- Previously he was first admitted to hospital for one month, at the age of 19 years, when he exhibited thought insertion, thought echo and delusions of reference. He had a well-established history of illicit drug abuse at this time and was subsequently diagnosed with a drug-induced psychosis. He responded to **chlorpromazine** 50 mg tds. This was continued for six months after discharge and then gradually reduced and stopped in the outpatient clinic by his consultant psychiatrist.
- He was re-admitted to hospital for two months at the age of 22 years, with a similar presentation to his first admission. However, in addition he exhibited persecutory delusions and formal thought disorder. He was no longer abusing illicit drugs at this time and was subsequently diagnosed with schizophrenia. He responded to the depot antipsychotic injection **zuclopenthixol decanoate** 300 mg once every two weeks and **procyclidine** 5 mg tds, both of which he was discharged on and complied with fully.
- He was recently reviewed in the outpatient clinic by his consultant psychiatrist, who felt that his recent deterioration represented a relapse of his schizophrenia with negative symptoms dominating the clinical picture.

What is the psychopharmacological management of this patient?

ANSWER 24

SCHIZOPHRENIA WITH NEGATIVE SYMPTOMS

- It is worth considering switching to a more alerting depot anti-psychotic injection – **flupenthixol decanoate** is useful in treating retarded or withdrawn schizophrenic patients in view of its apparent alerting nature; cf **zuclopenthixol decanoate,** which is not suitable for the treatment of retarded or withdrawn schizophrenic patients since it may exacerbate psychomotor retardation in such patients in view of its sedative nature.
- If the patient fails to respond to **flupenthixol decanoate** 400 mg weekly (maximum dose), it is worth considering switching to the world's first-ever atypical antipsychotic long-acting intramuscular (IM) injection, namely IM **risperidone.** This is licensed for the treatment of both the positive and the negative symptoms of schizophrenia and it also alleviates affective symptoms associated with schizophrenia.
- If the patient partially responds to IM **risperidone** 50 mg once every two weeks (maximum dose) it is worth considering adding in the oral atypical antipsychotic drug **amisulpride** – this is licensed for the treatment of schizophrenic patients with predominantly negative symptoms (dose range 50 mg to 300 mg daily, with an optimum dosage of 100 mg once a day).
- If the addition of **amisulpride** to IM **risperidone** proves ineffective it is worth considering a trial of the oral atypical antipsychotic drug **aripiprazole**; that is, stopping the **amisulpride** and substituting it with **aripiprazole,** which is then added to IM **risperidone.**

QUESTION 25

SCHIZOPHRENIFORM PSYCHOSIS IN A PATIENT WITH EPILEPSY

- A 32-year-old Caucasian man.
- He was taken to the police station by the police under Section 136 of the Mental Health Act 1983.
- A 10-year history of resistant temporal lobe epilepsy (complex partial seizures).
- He presented with threatening to kill his mother with a kitchen knife because of the persistent delusion that she was in communication with aliens who were collaborating with her to kill him.
- He exhibited persecutory delusions, audible thoughts, thought withdrawal and formal thought disorder.
- He was admitted to hospital and administered **chlorpromazine** 200 mg tds. He was subsequently diagnosed with a schizophreniform psychosis of epilepsy.
- His anti-epileptic medication on admission was **sodium valproate** 1.2 gram bd and **carbamazepine** 200 mg bd.
- Following admission, he was observed to have daily epileptic seizures (one a day) for the first week.
- The advice of a consultant neurologist was sought, and as a result his **carbamazepine** was gradually increased to 400 mg bd. His epileptic seizures subsequently stopped. In addition, his psychotic symptoms fully resolved in response to the **chlorpromazine.**
- The patient was subsequently discharged from hospital after a one-month period. The working diagnosis is that of an inter-ictal schizophreniform psychosis, that is, a schizophreniform psychosis occurring independently of epileptic seizures.

What is the psychopharmacological management of this patient?

ANSWER 25

SCHIZOPHRENIFORM PSYCHOSIS IN A PATIENT WITH EPILEPSY

- In inter-ictal schizophreniform psychosis, long-term antipsychotic treatment will probably be necessary.
- When choosing an antipsychotic drug in a patient with epilepsy, it is important to take into account what effects the antipsychotic has on lowering the seizure threshold and whether the antipsychotic is likely to interact with any anti-epileptic medication the patient is taking.
- In this patient, consider switching to an antipsychotic with a low pro-convulsive effect since **chlorpromazine** is one of the most epilepto-genic of the older conventional antipsychotic drugs.
- The conventional antipsychotic **haloperidol** would be a good choice in this patient. It has a low pro-convulsive effect. However, **carbamaze-pine** increases its rate of metabolism and larger doses of **haloperidol** may be required.
- If **haloperidol** proves unsuccessful, consider switching to the conventional antipsychotic **sulpiride**. It has a low pro-convulsive effect (albeit there is less clinical experience with **sulpiride**, cf **haloperidol**). In addition, **sulpiride** has no known interactions with anti-convulsants.
- If **sulpiride** proves unsuccessful, consider switching to the atypical antipsychotic **risperidone**. It has a low pro-convulsive effect (albeit there is limited clinical experience with **risperidone**, cf **haloperidol** and **sulpiride**). However, **carbamazepine** increases its rate of metabolism and larger doses of **risperidone** may be required.

QUESTION 26

SCHIZOPHRENIA IN PREGNANCY

- A 32-year-old Caucasian woman.
- She was admitted to hospital due to a deteriorating mental state.
- Presented with a three-week history of a gradual decline in her self-care, sleep disturbance, irritability and suspiciousness.
- She believed that her husband was going to poison her. She admitted to hearing two voices talking to each other about killing her and killing her baby (believing herself to be pregnant).
- She exhibited persecutory delusions, third-person auditory hallucinations and showed some evidence of self-neglect in that she was emaciated and unkempt.
- She had been diagnosed with schizophrenia 10 years ago on her first hospital admission. She has had two subsequent relapses, both of which were precipitated by non-compliance with oral antipsychotic medication (**chlorpromazine** the first time, **risperidone** the second time) as a result of adverse effects. During her last admission four years ago, she was prescribed the depot antipsychotic injection **pipotiazine palmitate** (formerly known as **pipothiazine palmitate**) 50 mg intramuscularly (IM) once every four weeks and **procyclidine** 5 mg twice daily, on which she has remained clinically stable up to her recent deterioration. She has remained compliant with her depot injection.
- The working diagnosis is that of a relapse of a schizophrenic illness.
- Following this admission to hospital a pregnancy test was done, which was positive. A subsequent ultrasound scan confirmed that she was approximately two months pregnant.

What is the psychopharmacological management of this patient?

ANSWER 26

SCHIZOPHRENIA IN PREGNANCY

- Depot antipsychotic injections should be avoided in the treatment of schizophrenia in pregnancy due to their prolonged action (making it difficult to adjust the doses) and their relatively high incidence of adverse effects, cf oral antipsychotic preparations.
- In this patient, consider switching to an oral conventional anti-psychotic drug owing to their safety data and because there is more clinical experience with them, cf oral atypical antipsychotic drugs.
- The conventional antipsychotic **haloperidol** would be a good choice in this patient. There has been widespread use of **haloperidol** in preg-nancy and it is recommended by some clinicians as the antipsychotic of choice.
- If the patient fails to respond to **haloperidol,** consider switching to the conventional antipsychotic **trifluoperazine.** It is one of the anti-psychotics with the most safety data in pregnancy. In addition, it is one of the antipsychotics with the most clinical experience.
- If the patient fails to respond to **trifluoperazine,** consider switching to the atypical antipsychotic **olanzapine.** It is one of the atypical anti-psychotics with the most data. In addition, it is widely used by peri-natal services in the UK.

QUESTION 27

SCHIZOAFFECTIVE DISORDER (SCHIZOMANIA)

- A 30-year-old Caucasian man.
- He was admitted to the acute general psychiatric ward of the local district general hospital from the Accident and Emergency Department.
- Presented with a one-month history of hearing two voices arguing with each other about him, the experience that others can 'read' his thoughts as they are 'broadcast' from his mind and the sensations of sexual intercourse attributed to unwanted sexual interference by a series of persecutors. In addition, he presented with the belief that he is a religious prophet and the experience of hearing a voice speaking to him about his special powers and expansive ideas, believing that his ideas are original, and that his work is of importance and of outstanding quality.
- He exhibited third-person auditory hallucinations, thought broadcasting, somatic hallucinations, grandiose delusions, second-person auditory hallucinations and expansive ideas. In addition, he exhibited a variation in his mood, with him at times displaying incongruity of affect, while at other times his mood was one of euphoria with infectious gaiety.
- He has an established diagnosis of schizoaffective disorder.
- This is his second episode of schizomania in the last 12 months.
- He experienced remission of his symptoms from his first episode of schizomania on the typical antipsychotic drug **haloperidol.** Unfortunately, he subsequently developed extra-pyramidal side-effects (EPSE) and **haloperidol** was then switched to the atypical antipsychotic drug **risperidone** six months ago.
- This episode of schizomania was precipitated by non-compliance with **risperidone,** which he stopped taking two months prior to admission owing to the side-effects of agitation and insomnia. The patient is now reluctant to take oral antipsychotic medication following his experience of side-effects on both **haloperidol** and **risperidone.**

What is the psychopharmacological management of this patient?

ANSWER 27

SCHIZOAFFECTIVE DISORDER (SCHIZOMANIA)

- An antipsychotic depot injection should now be considered for prophylaxis in view of the patient's reluctance to take oral antipsychotic medication.
- The antipsychotic depot injection of choice in such a patient who is poorly compliant with oral antipsychotic medication may be considered to be the conventional depot injection **pipotiazine palmitate** (formerly known as **pipothiazine palmitate**) – since this injection need only be administered once every four weeks and because it allegedly has few extra-pyramidal side-effects (EPSE), cf other conventional antipsychotic depot injections. **Pipotiazine palmitate** may also be considered in preference to intramuscular (IM) **risperidone,** the world's first-ever atypical antipsychotic long-acting IM injection – since IM **risperidone** is likely to cause the same side-effects of agitation and insomnia that the patient previously experienced on oral **risperidone.**
- Alongside the antipsychotic depot injection, an antimanic drug should also be considered for prophylaxis of schizoaffective disorder (schizomania).
- The antimanic drug of choice in such a patient who is reluctant to take oral medication may be considered to be **valproate semisodium*** – since this has low toxicity and regular serum level estimation appears to be unnecessary, cf **lithium carbonate,** which is a more toxic drug and does require regular serum level estimation.

* Used but this indication is not currently licensed in the UK.

QUESTION 28

ACUTE ORGANIC DISORDER

- A 20-year-old Caucasian woman.
- She presented to the Accident and Emergency Department of the local teaching hospital with an acute onset and fluctuating course of impairment of consciousness recognised by slowness, uncertainty about the time of day and poor concentration. Her behaviour took the form of inactivity, slowness and repetitive purposeless movements.
- She exhibited reduced speech and a mood of anxiety, irritability, depression and agitation. Her thoughts were slow and muddled but rich in content. She had ideas of reference and persecutory delusions that were transient and poorly elaborated. She also exhibited visual illusions, visual misinterpretations and visual hallucinations with a fantastic content. In addition, she exhibited depersonalisation and de-realisation. With regard to cognition, she was disorientated in time and place, and had disturbance of memory affecting registration, retention, recall and new learning. Her insight was impaired.
- She was on no prescribed medication.
- There is no past psychiatric history.
- The working diagnosis is that of a first episode of an acute organic disorder (delirium).

What are the possible causes of this first episode of delirium?
What is the management of this patient?

ANSWER 28

ACUTE ORGANIC DISORDER

The aetiology (possible causes) of this acute organic disorder may be considered as follows.

1 Alcohol/drugs:
   (a) Alcohol or other drug intoxication (e.g. L-dopa, anticholinergics, anxiolytics – hypnotics, anti-convulsants, opiates).
   (b) Withdrawal of alcohol or other drugs.
2 Metabolic causes:
   (a) Uraemia.
   (b) Electrolyte imbalance (e.g. hypercalcaemia).
   (c) Cardiac failure.
   (d) Respiratory failure.
   (e) Hepatic failure.
   (f) Acute intermittent porphyria.
   (g) Systemic lupus erythematosus (SLE).
3 Endocrine causes:
   (a) Hyperthyroidism.
   (b) Hypothyroidism.
   (c) Hypoparathyroidism.
   (d) Hypopituitarism.
   (e) Hypoglycaemia.
4 Infective causes:
   (a) Intercranial infection:
       – Encephalitis.
       – Meningitis.
   (b) Systemic infection:
       – Septicaemia.
       – Pneumonia.
5 Other intra-cranial lesions:
   (a) Space occupying lesion.
   (b) Raised intra-cranial pressure.
6 Vitamin deficiency:
   (a) B_1 (Thiamine) – Wernicke's encephalopathy.
   (b) B_{12}.
   (c) Nicotinic acid.
7 Head injury
8 Heavy metals:
   (a) Heavy metal intoxication (e.g. lead, manganese).
9 Epilepsy.

The management of this acute organic disorder may be considered as follows.

1 Specific measures:
   (a) The fundamental treatment is directed to the physical cause.
   (b) In some cases – the effect of appropriate treatment is quite immediate and dramatic, and little more treatment is required, e.g. in the case of hypoglycaemia.
   (c) In most cases – recovery is more protracted and it is important to observe certain general measures.
2 General measures:
   (a) The patient should be nursed in a well-lit room, preferably a side ward.
   (b) Medical and nursing staff should reassure the patient, and explain to her both where she is and what is the purpose of any examination or treatment.
   (c) The patient should be comfortable, adequately hydrated and in electrolyte balance.
3 Drug treatment:
   (a) During the daytime:
       – It may be necessary to calm the patient without inducing drowsiness.
       – The drug of choice is **haloperidol**, which calms without causing drowsiness and postural hypotension, cf **chlorpromazine**.
       – The effective daily dose of **haloperidol** usually varies from 10 mg to 30 mg.
   (b) At night:
       – It may be necessary to help the patient sleep.
       – A suitable drug is a sedative anxiolytic drug (i.e. a benzodiazepine), which promotes sleep.
   (c) In the special case of hepatic failure – benzodiazepines may be used during the daytime despite their sedative effects, since they are less likely to precipitate coma, cf **haloperidol** (which is the usual drug of choice to calm such patients).
   (d) In the special case of alcohol withdrawal – **chlordiazepoxide** is a suitable drug.

QUESTION 29

ALZHEIMER'S DISEASE (MILD TO MODERATE)

- A 78-year-old Caucasian man.
- He was admitted to the old-age psychiatric ward of the local teaching hospital following a domiciliary visit by a consultant in old-age psychiatry.
- He presented with a six-month history of increasing forgetfulness, deterioration in self-care and deterioration in personal hygiene. He also presented with changes in his behaviour in the form of episodes of restlessness and wandering at night, aggression and sexual disinhibition. In addition, he presented with depressive symptoms in the form of feeling depressed, appetite loss, weight loss and sleep disturbance.
- He exhibited cognitive impairment in the form of loss of memory for recent events and disorientation in time. His mood was depressed.
- There is no past psychiatric history.
- There is a family psychiatric history of dementia in that both of his parents have been diagnosed with dementia.
- The working diagnosis is that of Alzheimer's disease (mild to moderate) associated with behavioural symptoms of dementia and accompanied by depressive symptoms.

What is the psychopharmacological management of this patient?

ANSWER 29

ALZHEIMER'S DISEASE (MILD TO MODERATE)

- Acetylcholinesterase-inhibiting drugs are used in the treatment of Alzheimer's disease, specifically for mild to moderate disease. From this group of drugs, **donepezil** may be considered to be the best tolerated and it may also be considered to have the simplest dosage regimen, with an initial dose of 5 mg once daily at bedtime, increased if necessary after one month to 10 mg daily (the maximum dose). **Donepezil** was the first drug to be licensed in the UK for the treatment of mild to moderate dementia in Alzheimer's disease.
- Treatment with drugs for dementia should be initiated and supervised only by a specialist experienced in the management of dementia. The evidence to support the use of these drugs relates to their cognitive enhancement. Benefit is assessed by repeating the cognitive assessment at around three months after initiating treatment. Such cognitive assessment cannot demonstrate how the disease may have progressed in the absence of treatment, but it can give a good guide to the response to treatment. As many as half of the patients administered acetylcholinesterase-inhibiting drugs will demonstrate a slower rate of cognitive decline. The drug should be discontinued in those thought not to be responding to medication. Many specialists repeat the cognitive assessment four to six weeks after discontinuation of medication to assess deterioration in cognitive functioning. If significant deterioration in cognitive functioning occurs during this short period, consideration should be given to restarting drug therapy.
- Atypical antipsychotic drugs are used in the treatment of the behavioural symptoms of dementia. These are preferable to typical (conventional) antipsychotic drugs, which may worsen cognitive decline in dementia. Among the atypical antipsychotic drugs, **olanzapine** and **risperidone** are associated with an increased risk of stroke in elderly patients with dementia. As a consequence, the Committee on Safety of Medicines (CSM) has advised that **risperidone** and **olanzapine** should not be used for treating behavioural symptoms of dementia. From the remainder of the atypicals, **quetiapine** may be considered to be the atypical antipsychotic of choice to treat behavioural disturbance in dementia. Since the imposition of restrictions on the use of **risperidone** and **olanzapine**, **quetiapine** has become widely used at a dose of 50 mg to 100 mg daily. Apart from **quetiapine**, **amisulpride** is also considered quite efficacious as an atypical antipsychotic drug used in the treatment of the behavioural symptoms of dementia.
- To alleviate depressive symptoms, a trial of antidepressant medication is worthwhile, even in the presence of dementia. Tricyclic antidepressants (TCAs) tend to increase confusion in the elderly owing to anti-cholinergic side-effects – therefore selective serotonin reuptake

inhibitors (SSRIs) may be regarded as the first-line antidepressant therapy of choice in this patient. From the SSRIs, taking into account safety and tolerability, **sertraline** and **citalopram** may be considered to be the preferred antidepressants since both may have a lower potential for drug interactions as a consequence of their both having no significant interaction with cytochrome P450 2D6.

QUESTION 30

ANOREXIA NERVOSA

- A 19-year-old Caucasian woman.
- She was referred by her general practitioner to a specialist eating disorder unit for a psychiatric opinion.
- Presented with a body weight more than 25% below the standard weight, a body mass index (BMI – calculated as weight in kilograms divided by the square of the height in metres) of less than 17.5, an intense wish to be thin and amenorrhoea (as a primary symptom). She also presented with the central psychological features of a fear of being fat, a relentless pursuit of a low body weight and a distorted image of her body – believing herself to be too fat even when severely under-weight. In addition, she presented with anxiety, agitation and depressive symptoms. Psychotic features were also present as a complication of starvation.
- Her pursuit of thinness took several forms, with her generally eating very little and showing a particular avoidance of carbohydrates. She also tried to achieve the pursuit of thinness by inducing vomiting, excessive exercise and purging. In addition, she also had episodes of uncontrollable overeating (binge eating or bulimia); after overeating she would feel bloated and might induce vomiting. Such binges were followed by remorse and intensified efforts to lose weight.
- She exhibited clinical features secondary to starvation in the form of sensitivity to cold, constipation, low blood pressure, bradycardia, hypothermia and lanugo hair (hair on the trunk). She also exhibited physical consequences secondary to vomiting and laxative abuse in the form of hypokalaemia. In addition, she exhibited hormonal abnormalities in the form of an elevated prolactin level and a reduced oestradiol level.
- Delayed gastric emptying was also evident, as was impairment of colonic functioning caused by chronic laxative abuse.
- Her parents described her as being a happy child until they separated when she was 12 years old. She subsequently coped poorly with puberty and became increasingly preoccupied with food.
- A working diagnosis of anorexia nervosa was made by the consultant psychiatrist in the specialist eating disorder unit and she was admitted for further assessment.

What is the psychopharmacological management of this patient?

ANSWER 30

ANOREXIA NERVOSA

- Any psychopharmacological interventions for her anorexia nervosa must take into account her primary problem of a low body mass index (BMI) in addition to her secondary physical complications.
- With regard to her psychotic symptoms, anxiety and agitation, an antipsychotic drug may be considered for treatment. When choosing a suitable antipsychotic drug in this patient, it is important to consider one with minimal potential to prolong the QT_c interval – since the patient has hypokalaemia (as a physical consequence secondary to vomiting and laxative abuse) which in itself may lead to prolongation of the QT_c interval. This, in turn, is thought to be a risk factor for the development of ventricular arrhythmias and sudden death.
- It is also important to consider an antipsychotic drug with minimal potential to elevate the prolactin level – since the patient already has hyperprolactinaemia as well as a reduced oestradiol level (both as a physical consequence of her anorexia nervosa), which are both thought to be risk factors for the development of osteoporosis.
- Whilst an antipsychotic drug may be used to promote weight gain due to its side-effect profile, and this might appear advantageous superficially, in clinical practice such drug-induced weight gain is likely to be unacceptable to the patient and therefore may have a negative effect on her future compliance with medication as well as on the future progress of her anorexia nervosa.
- Having considered all of the above issues, the atypical antipsychotic drug **aripiprazole** may be considered as the first-line antipsychotic drug of choice in this patient – since it is not associated with ECG changes and therefore has no requirement for routine ECG monitoring. Moreover, it is associated with a prolactin level comparable with placebo and has minimal weight gain due to low affinity for serotonin $5HT_{2c}$ receptors.
- With regard to her depressive symptoms, an antidepressant drug may be considered for treatment. Although antidepressants may be used theoretically to promote weight gain because of their side-effect profile, there is little evidence to support their use in anorexia nervosa to increase the rate of weight gain. The selective serotonin reuptake inhibitors (SSRIs) may be considered as the antidepressant group of choice in this patient – there is evidence that they may be effective in relapse prevention after weight restoration in patients with anorexia nervosa; there is also evidence that such patients show an improvement in mood, a reduction in eating disorder symptoms and a reduction in obsessionality. In addition, unlike tricyclic antidepressants (TCAs), SSRIs are less likely to exacerbate constipation in patients with anorexia nervosa.

- With regard to her hypokalaemia, it is important to correct this electrolyte disturbance. Oral therapy is preferred – if potassium levels are restored to normal too rapidly there is a risk of dangerous depletion of phosphate, calcium and magnesium. If possible, dietary replacement of potassium with potassium-rich foods may suffice (e.g. bananas).
- With regard to her delayed gastric emptying, **domperidone** may be considered preferable as it does not cross the blood–brain barrier, cf **metoclopramide**.
- With regard to her chronic laxative abuse, resulting in impairment of colonic functioning, the occasional stimulant **or** osmotic laxative may be considered.

QUESTION 31

ACUTE ALCOHOL WITHDRAWAL/ALCOHOL DEPENDENCE

- A 48-year-old Caucasian man.
- He was referred from the Accident and Emergency Department of the local teaching hospital for a psychiatric opinion.
- Following cessation of heavy drinking (one and a half bottles of spirits a day for the last few weeks), he presented with a 48-hour history of general withdrawal symptoms from alcohol in the form of acute tremulousness affecting the hands, legs and trunk ('the shakes'), agitation, nausea, retching, sweating and perceptual distortions. In addition, he presented with tactile, auditory and visual hallucinations and convulsions.
- He subsequently went on to exhibit delirium tremens, the fully developed withdrawal syndrome from alcohol in the form of clouding of consciousness, disorientation in time and place, impairment of recent memory, illusions, tactile, auditory and visual hallucinations (particularly of diminutive people and animals – 'Lilliputian' hallucinations), persecutory delusions, agitation and restlessness, fearful affect, prolonged insomnia, tremulous hands, trunkal ataxia and autonomic over-activity.
- He has a well-established diagnosis of alcohol dependence, displaying a subjective awareness of compulsion to drink, a stereotyped pattern of drinking, an increased tolerance to alcohol, primacy of drinking over other activities, repeated withdrawal symptoms, relief drinking and reinstatement after abstinence. He has been heavily dependent on alcohol for the last 20 years and has incurred physical damage to his liver as demonstrated by highly elevated liver function tests (LFTs).
- He has had four admissions for inpatient detoxification from alcohol in the last three years prior to presentation. He has also undergone four community detoxifications through a specialist alcohol day hospital attached to the teaching hospital in the previous six years. Previous detoxifications have been uncomplicated, with the exception of one grand mal seizure which occurred 48 hours into his most recent admission to hospital six months ago. He has previously attempted controlled drinking unsuccessfully.
- The working diagnosis is that of acute alcohol withdrawal in the setting of an established diagnosis of alcohol dependence.

What is the psychopharmacological management of this patient?

ANSWER 31

ACUTE ALCOHOL WITHDRAWAL/ALCOHOL DEPENDENCE

- Delirium tremens is a medical emergency requiring early diagnosis and an urgent transfer to an inpatient medical setting. This setting allows for the safe administration of intravenous **diazepam** to treat any convulsions and also for the safe administration of parenteral **thiamine** since the patient is at high risk of developing symptoms of Wernicke's encephalopathy. Inpatient medical care is also the most appropriate environment for the patient to receive fluid and electrolyte replacement to correct any electrolyte imbalance and to receive glucose to correct any hypoglycaemia. Antibiotics could also be safely administered to treat any infection. A full medical assessment of the patient is required.
- Detoxification of the patient is also required, that is, management of the general withdrawal symptoms from alcohol. This involves sedation using the long-acting benzodiazepines **clomethiazole (chlormethiazole)** or **chlordiazepoxide** – these sedative drugs are generally prescribed to attenuate withdrawal symptoms but they also have a dependence potential. To minimise this risk of dependence, administration should be for a limited period only, for example **chlordiazepoxide** 10 mg to 50 mg qds gradually reducing over 7 to 14 days. Benzodiazepines should not be prescribed if the patient is likely to continue drinking alcohol. Moreover, if **clomethiazole** is taken in combination with alcohol, each potentiates the central nervous system (CNS) depressant action of the other, and overdosage is frequently fatal; thus, nowadays **chlordiazepoxide** is preferred to **clomethiazole**.
- Once detoxified, the patient's mental state should be reassessed to establish whether or not there is any underlying clinical depression – if present, treatment of the underlying disorder should be considered using one of the selective serotonin reuptake inhibitors (SSRIs), since they appear to have no clinically significant interaction with alcohol. In addition, there is some evidence that SSRIs reduce alcohol craving and alcohol consumption in patients with alcohol dependence; however, the results of studies to date have been rather disappointing.
- Once the patient is detoxified, pharmacological treatment for the maintenance of abstinence should be considered. **Acamprosate,** which works on the gaba/glutamate system, is licensed in the UK for maintenance of abstinence and may be considered as the drug of choice for this therapeutic indication. It reduces alcohol craving, is non-addictive, does not interact with alcohol and is associated with relatively few side-effects. In combination with relapse prevention

counselling, **acamprosate** may be helpful in maintaining abstinence in alcohol-dependent patients. It should be initiated as soon as possible after abstinence from alcohol has been achieved and should be maintained if the patient relapses. However, if the patient continues to abuse alcohol, this negates the therapeutic benefits of **acamprosate.** NB: *Acamprosate cannot be used when there is very significant hepatic damage.*

- Other pharmacological treatments for the maintenance of abstinence after detoxification include:

  (a) **Disulfiram** – an aversive stimulant, inducing nausea in the patient if alcohol is consumed; efficacy limited by problems with compliance (patients who wish to start drinking again tend to stop the **disulfiram** to avoid the nausea).

  (b) **Naltrexone*** – an opiate receptor antagonist; licensed in the USA for the maintenance of abstinence.

- Total abstinence is a better goal-orientated treatment plan for the drinking problem in this patient, since he is over 40, is heavily dependent on alcohol, has incurred physical damage and has previously attempted controlled drinking unsuccessfully, cf controlled drinking as the goal-orientated treatment plan.

* Used but this indication is not currently licensed in the UK.

QUESTION 32

ACUTE OPIATE WITHDRAWAL/CHRONIC OPIATE DEPENDENCE

- A 28-year-old Caucasian man.
- He was referred from the Accident and Emergency Department of the local district general hospital for a psychiatric opinion.
- Following cessation of heavy heroin abuse (smoking 1 gram of heroin per day for the last four weeks) he presented with a 36-hour history of withdrawal effects from opiates in the form of piloerection, shivering, abdominal cramps, diarrhoea, lacrimation, rhinorrhoea, dilated pupils, tachycardia, yawning, intense craving for heroin, agitation and restlessness.
- He exhibited clinical features of chronic opiate dependence in the form of constipation, constricted pupils, chronic malaise, weakness, impotence and tremors.
- He has a well-established history of heroin dependence, displaying both psychic and physical dependence. He started to smoke heroin at the age of 18 and began smoking it daily from the age of 27. Previously, he has been referred by his general practitioner to the local drug service, which initiated him on **methadone**, the dose of which was gradually increased up to 60 mg (60 ml) daily to cover withdrawal symptoms from heroin. He was monitored by the local drug service for a period of six months and managed to remain off street heroin during this time. However, he subsequently disengaged from the service about 12 months ago and returned to smoking street heroin.
- The working diagnosis is that of acute opiate withdrawal in the setting of an established diagnosis of chronic opiate dependence.

What is the psychopharmacological management of this patient?

ANSWER 32

ACUTE OPIATE WITHDRAWAL/CHRONIC OPIATE DEPENDENCE

Detoxification of the patient is required in the first instance, that is, management of the withdrawal effects from opiates. This can be done in several ways.

1 Using **methadone** (an opioid agonist) given as a mixture in a reducing dosage regimen. Initially the patient is prescribed 10 mg to 40 mg of **methadone** daily; this may be increased by up to 10 mg daily (with a maximum weekly increase of 30 mg) until there are no signs of opiate withdrawal or intoxication evident (usual dose range of **methadone** required is 60 mg to 120 mg daily). The dosage of the **methadone** is then gradually decreased and stopped. Such a reducing dosage regimen is nearly always undertaken as an outpatient (through the local drug service).

NB: *To help the patient to reduce his* **methadone** *from doses of 20 mg (20 ml) or less down to zero, a 21-day* **lofexidine** *regimen may be used; blood pressure should be monitored twice a week.*

2 Using **buprenorphine** (an opioid partial agonist) given by sublingual administration. It may be used as an alternative substitute treatment to **methadone** for patients with moderate opioid dependence. **Buprenorphine** has a milder withdrawal syndrome than **methadone** and thus may be the preferred substitution therapy for detoxification programmes for patients with moderate opioid dependence (and greater potential for abuse).
3 Symptomatic relief using **chlorpromazine** and analgesics – an option but generally not the preferred choice in clinical practice.

Once detoxified, pharmacological treatment for the maintenance of abstinence should be considered. **Naltrexone** (an opioid antagonist) is licensed in the UK for the maintenance of abstinence. In combination with relapse prevention counselling, **naltrexone** may be helpful in maintaining abstinence in opiate-dependent patients. It should be initiated in a specialist drug clinic only once the patient has completed detoxification; that is, as soon as possible after abstinence from opiates has been achieved. The starting dose is half a tablet (25 mg) in the morning on day one. From then onwards, the dose is one tablet (50 mg) in the morning for up to six months. If the patient continues to abuse opiates while taking **naltrexone** regularly, he will not experience euphoria. This is because the euphoric reaction of opioid agonists is blocked by **naltrexone** (owing to its being an opioid antagonist). NB: *It is vital to monitor liver function tests (LFTs) closely, at least in the early stages of treatment with* **naltrexone***.*

QUESTION 33

ACUTE BENZODIAZEPINE WITHDRAWAL/CHRONIC BENZODIAZEPINE DEPENDENCE

- A 35-year-old Caucasian lady.
- She was referred from the Accident and Emergency Department of the local district general hospital for a psychiatric opinion.
- Following cessation of heavy **lorazepam** abuse (12 mg of oral **lorazepam** daily in divided doses for the last few weeks) she presented with a 24-hour history of withdrawal effects from benzodiazepines in the form of rebound insomnia, tremor, anxiety, restlessness, appetite disturbance, weight loss, sweating, convulsions, confusion, toxic psychosis and a condition resembling delirium tremens (the fully developed withdrawal syndrome from alcohol).
- She exhibited clinical features of chronic benzodiazepine dependence in the form of unsteadiness of gait, dysarthria, drowsiness and nystagmus.
- She has a well-established history of benzodiazepine dependence, displaying both psychic and physical dependence. She started to take oral **lorazepam** at the age of 28 years and began taking it daily from the age of 30. She was previously prescribed 15 mg of oral **diazepam** daily, in divided doses, by her general practitioner for a period of six months and managed to remain off **lorazepam** during this time. However, she subsequently disengaged from this treatment regimen about 12 months ago and returned to **lorazepam** abuse.
- The working diagnosis is that of acute benzodiazepine withdrawal in the setting of an established diagnosis of chronic benzodiazepine dependence.

What is the psychopharmacological management of this patient?

ANSWER 33

ACUTE BENZODIAZEPINE WITHDRAWAL/CHRONIC BENZODIAZEPINE DEPENDENCE

- A condition resembling delirium tremens is a medical emergency requiring early diagnosis and an urgent transfer to an inpatient medical setting. This setting allows for the safe administration of intravenous (IV) **diazepam** to treat any convulsions. A full medical assessment of the patient is required in this setting.
- Detoxification of the patient is also required, that is, management of the withdrawal effects from benzodiazepines. This involves switching the patient from the current short-acting benzodiazepine **lorazepam** to the long-acting benzodiazepine **diazepam.** The rationale for this transfer is that it is considered easier to withdraw a patient from a long-acting benzodiazepine, cf a short-acting benzodiazepine. Such detoxification may be undertaken either as an outpatient or as an inpatient.
- Once the patient has been successfully switched from **lorazepam** to **diazepam**, the dosage of **diazepam** should be gradually decreased, and eventually the **diazepam** should be stopped.
- There is some evidence to support the use of antidepressant medication as an adjunctive treatment to cover the withdrawal symptoms from the **diazepam** as this is gradually being withdrawn. A suitable choice for such an antidepressant drug would be one with sedative and anxiolytic properties, such as **dosulepin** (formerly known as **dothiepin**) at a starting dose of 75 mg nocte, increased after four days to 150 mg nocte.
- Once the **diazepam** has been stopped, the dosage of **dosulepin** should be gradually decreased, and eventually the **dosulepin** should be stopped. Relapse prevention counselling for the maintenance of abstinence should also be considered following detoxification of the patient from benzodiazepines.

QUESTION 34

SELF-INJURIOUS BEHAVIOUR (SIB)/LEARNING DISABILITY/TEMPORAL LOBE EPILEPSY

- A 25-year-old Caucasian man.
- He was referred from the Accident and Emergency Department of the local district general hospital for a psychiatric opinion.
- Presented with a one-month history of increasing self-injurious behaviour (SIB) in the form of head banging, banging other body parts, face beating, biting himself on his knees and his shoulders, eye gouging, pulling his own hair, skin picking, scratching, slapping himself, smashing windows using his hands, pinching himself and pica (i.e. eating things which are not food, such as faeces, plastic, dirt and stones).
- He also presented with a one-month history of increasing anti-social behaviours in the form of screaming, shouting and faecal smearing as well as increasingly aggressive outbursts against both property and other people (e.g. ripping his bedding and his clothes, biting others and trying to pull back the fingers of others).
- In addition, he presented with a one-month history of atypical depressive symptoms in the form of sleeping excessively, increased appetite, increased weight and diurnal variation in mood (his mood being worse in the evening) as well as anxiety, phobic anxiety, obsessional and hypochondriacal symptoms.
- The patient has a past psychiatric history of a learning disability, the cause of which is unknown.
- The patient also has a past psychiatric history of temporal lobe epilepsy (complex partial seizures) controlled with **phenytoin**. However, in the last month he has suffered side-effects on this medication in the form of nausea, vomiting and constipation, which have resulted in his partial compliance with the **phenytoin**. This, in turn, appears to have resulted in him suffering with a couple of complex partial seizures in the last month.
- The working diagnosis is that of SIB in the context of an established diagnosis of a learning disability and temporal lobe epilepsy.

What is the psychopharmacological management of this patient?

ANSWER 34

SELF-INJURIOUS BEHAVIOUR (SIB)/LEARNING DISABILITY/TEMPORAL LOBE EPILEPSY

- It appears that the patient has displayed intolerable side-effects to the anti-convulsant **phenytoin,** resulting in poor compliance with medication and increased seizure activity. As a consequence of this, a change in anti-epileptic medication should be considered.
- **Carbamazepine** may be considered to be the anti-convulsant of choice to switch to in this patient – it is generally regarded as the drug of choice for temporal lobe epilepsy (complex partial seizures). It has generally fewer side-effects than **phenytoin**. Moreover, it has a wider therapeutic index than **phenytoin** and the relationship between dose and plasma **carbamazepine** concentration is linear. There is also some evidence that **carbamazepine** may reduce self-injurious behaviour (SIB) in patients with learning disability. In addition, there is some evidence that **carbamazepine** may be useful in the treatment of aggressive behaviour.
- Antipsychotic drugs should be used with caution in this patient when considering them for the treatment of SIB or behavioural disturbances due to their lowering of the convulsive threshold and subsequent potential for increasing seizure activity.
- An antidepressant should be considered to treat the depressive symptoms. The reversible inhibitor of monoamine oxidase type A (RIMA) **moclobemide** may be considered to be the antidepressant of choice in this patient – it is indicated in the treatment of atypical depressive disorders and there is no caution for its use in patients with epilepsy, cf other antidepressant drugs.
- Consider involving the advice of a specialist neurologist.

QUESTION 35

THE ACUTELY DISTURBED PATIENT – RAPID TRANQUILLISATION

- A 23-year-old Caucasian man.
- He was taken to the Custody Suite of the local police station having been detained by the police under Section 136 of the Mental Health Act 1983. He was found running naked down the street and became verbally abusive and physically aggressive when he was approached by a policeman. He was reported by the policeman to be speaking incoherently, using words he invented himself. Following assessment by a consultant psychiatrist, a second Section 12(2) approved medical practitioner and the duty social worker, he was subsequently admitted to the acute psychiatric unit of the local psychiatric hospital under Section 2 of the Mental Health Act 1983 for further assessment.
- He presented at hospital in an acutely disturbed manner directing verbal abuse and physical aggression towards the nursing staff.
- He exhibited neologisms. He also exhibited second-person auditory hallucinations taking the form of voices telling him to kill himself.
- The nursing staff adopted the strategy that much could be done for him by providing a calm, reassuring and consistent environment in which provocation was avoided. The patient was nursed in a special ward area with an adequate number of experienced staff in an attempt to avoid the use of heavy medication.
- There is no past psychiatric history or past forensic history.
- There is no family psychiatric history.
- The working diagnosis is that of an acutely disturbed patient where the underlying cause has yet to be determined.

What is the psychopharmacological management of this patient that is required to bring their acutely disturbed behaviour under immediate control?

ANSWER 35

THE ACUTELY DISTURBED PATIENT – RAPID TRANQUILLISATION

- In the first instance, oral medication should be offered to the patient. Since the patient is displaying psychotic symptoms, it is reasonable to consider an oral antipsychotic drug as first-line treatment.
- Historically, **haloperidol** has been the antipsychotic of choice in acutely disturbed behaviour. Up to 15 mg of **haloperidol** may be given orally in divided doses. However, in recent years the atypical antipsychotic **olanzapine** has been licensed for use in the management of the acutely disturbed patient. Up to 20 mg of **olanzapine** may be given orally daily in divided doses. **Olanzapine** has the advantage over **haloperidol** of being available as an orodispersible formulation ('velo-tab'), which is easier to take and more difficult to spit out than conventional tablets. **Olanzapine** also has the advantage over **halo-peridol** as being less likely to cause both extra-pyramidal side-effects (EPSE) and prolongation of the QT_c interval. Thus, **olanzapine** may now be considered to be the antipsychotic drug of choice in the management of the acutely disturbed patient.
- If response to an oral antipsychotic drug alone is insufficient, consider adding in the benzodiazepine **lorazepam*** in oral form. Up to 4 mg of **lorazepam** may be given orally daily in divided doses.
- If three doses of a combined oral antipsychotic and oral **lorazepam** are insufficient or if the patient refuses oral medication, consider administering the antipsychotic medication alone by the intramuscular (IM) route. Up to 18 mg of **haloperidol** may be given IM daily in divided doses for emergency control. Up to 20 mg of **olanzapine** may be given IM daily in divided doses for emergency control, with a recommended initial dose of 10 mg and the option of giving a second IM injection, 5 mg to 10 mg, two hours later. The maximum dose of IM **olanzapine** is 20 mg in 24 hours on three consecutive days.
- If IM **haloperidol** alone fails to bring the situation under control, the patient may be given in addition a slow IM injection of 2 mg of **lorazepam**,* if necessary repeated two hours later (i.e. up to 4 mg of IM **lorazepam** may be given daily in divided doses in combination with intramuscular **haloperidol**).
- If IM **olanzapine** alone fails to bring the situation under control, the patient may be given in addition a slowly delivered IM injection of 2 mg of **lorazepam**,* administered at a minimum of one hour after the administration of intramuscular **olanzapine**, cf IM **haloperidol**, which can be administered concurrently with IM **lorazepam**. Up to 4 mg of

* Used but this indication is not currently licensed in the UK.

intramuscular **lorazepam** may be given daily in divided doses in combination with IM **olanzapine.**

- If repeated IM injections of a combined antipsychotic and **lorazepam** are insufficient, consider the short-acting IM depot injection **zuclo-penthixol acetate,** which should be more easily administered to the patient. This can be given as a single injection at the maximum dose of 150 mg (dose range of 50 mg to 150 mg per injection). This may be repeated after two to three days (one additional dose may be needed one to two days after the first injection). The maximum cumulative dose is 400 mg per course of injections. A maximum of four injections may be given with a maximum duration of treatment of two weeks.

Index